Surrender To Heal

To order more books contact Sameboat,Inc.
www.Sameboat.tv www.
surrendertoheal.com or
the author at reggiesmith770@yahoo.com

REGGIE
SMITH

SURRENDER
TO HEAL

SEVEN WAYS TO RISE
ABOVE THE BATTLEFIELDS
OF LIFE

SAMEBOAT, INC.
2004

Surrender To Heal

Disclaimer

Names used are not real. Any similarity
to anyone living or dead is purely coinci-
dental. This is my story from my perspective and I am sticking to it. Nothing
derogatory is meant or implied.

TABLE OF CONTENTS

ACKNOWLEDGMENTS

There are many people who have contributed to my life and made valuable information available. I have been blessed to be exposed to many different schools of thought and learning opportunities. I appreciate them all and I attribute my opportunities for evolution to having learned something from them all. Of all these vessels of information and knowledge, my wife Dionne has been a great teacher, and she creates a fertile atmosphere for learning and the space for me to do so. She has stood with me throughout and has been my best friend. I love her very much, and this book is dedicated to her.

My mother Ethel Louise ("Lou") Smith has been a wonderful mother for my lovely sister Pamela and I. She has showered me with love and wisdom. She motivated me to be who I am, and allowed me, in the way any "Jewish mother" would, to live my own life. She has worked behind the scenes to help make things smooth for the family. She has, In her matter-of-fact kind of way, she has shared her wisdom with the entire family and me. My mother has protected me, counseled me and loved me like only a mother could. Her example of courage, strength, wisdom and dedication is one that I attempt to emulate. She is a very special person and words could never do justice to express my gratitude. I love you and hope that you are proud.

My dear departed father, Leroy Smith, who planted the

seed from which I have grown, thank you. As you used to say, "The apple doesn't fall far from the tree." I have been blessed to have had the opportunity to have your genes and to have known you. Your wit, intelligence, and complex nature provided me with what I needed in order to navigate the system of life. I remember you always. I wish you were here, but that would change God's story.

Pamela has been a gentle strength that I have often needed as a model. Her love has been unconditional and is reciprocated. She, too, has benefited from our experiences as children as exhibited by the loving, giving and unselfish person she has become. In my opinion, she, like my mother, is among the most selfless people I know. Pam has been supportive and loving at every stage of my life. I am glad to have you and your family in my life.

My oldest natural son, Jason, and in a different way his deceased brother Erin, have provided immense inspiration for me to go on when it seemed much easier to quit. Jason has been the mirror, looking glass and the prism with which I see life. I admire the man he has become and am honored to have had our experiences. Erin has proved it did not have to be.

I love you.

My beautiful daughter Jonell, and younger sons, Jamar and Jarod, are all loving, funny, intelligent manifestations of the relationship that I have had with God and their mother. I am blessed with their love and proud of who they are. We have been a true family and it has been a wonderful adventure we are having. The people they are inspire me.

I also have had some great master teachers in my life. They have been guides in this journey through this jungle. My spiritual guru, the deceased Maharaj Charan Singh Ji, and his successor Gurinder Singh Ji, have been the leaders of the spiritual path that has been my practice since I was exposed to it in 1987. The disciplines of that path have surely saved this mortal coil and continue to shape the experience of my spirit.

My relationship with Suzanne and Muhammad Zahir has been magical, filled with love, and the flashpoint of other wonderful relationships and synchronistic events that have led to a great wealth of knowledge and memories. Through them I have met and been taught consciousness and energy by Ramtha. As a team we attended IBI, an entrepreneur networking forum where I had a life-changing experience. I have been taught cooperative business and given the courage and opportunity to practice it while being what I believe God would have me be. I love them both dearly for their love, friendship and encouragement.

I have much respect and gratitude for my ex-wife and first girlfriend, Anne. She survived my addiction and showed me love and understanding. She weathered some of the hardest years of my life and has been a wonderful mother to my son Jason.

There have been so many people that have been instrumental in my "recovery" and to illuminating the journey of my life. I am sure that I will forget some, but I would like to acknowledge George and Ollie Johnson, Wayne Johnson, The Inwood Street Family, The Barfield Family, especially Mrs. Charlotte Barfield and The Whitman Family. My great friends Joe Pollack, Al Smith, and Steve Hunt really put their money where their hearts are. The Heavyhitters, Dr. William Richardson, Dr. Barbara Justice, and the many others who played a part in my being able to be, deserve my gratitude, and I give it to them freely.

Thanks, my falsely incarcerated Brother Aqyil Muhammad, for being an inspiration and showing me that there is true freedom in surrendering to what is. Thanks to his parents Carolyn and Maurice Donovan for providing their hospitality in their home in St.Thomas.

Aziz Saboor has been a brother, partner and motivator. He has been instrumental in the completion of this book. Aziz has been a big part of my personal evolution. His confidence and his fervent yet patient belief in the need for us to tell this story has given me the strength to do it. His passion for being a part of creating opportunities for the world to begin "having the conversation" and "participating in our own survival" has been instrumental. Aziz has been my friend and confidant and has financially helped my family and I to be able to do this and other works. He is very generous and I appreciate his being the reflection of our purpose. Thank you very much.

Thanks to Mr. Alton Taylor, my elder, neighbor and fellow author who gave me loving counsel and served a vessel for God to give me the message of write what you know about.

Thank God I am alive and thanks to all that have contributed to the idea that has become this book. Peace and blessings to all who have died as casualties in the war against alcoholism and AIDS.
A SPECIAL DEDICATION TO MY MOTHER AND FATHER whom have been the vessel for my life.

INTRODUCTION

This book is my attempt to be a vessel of God's word and an instrument of Her Will. I believe in a loving God as She/He may express itself through all things. I pray that these words will serve to stimulate a psychic change in the minds and hearts of those who are dealing with the diseases of addictions, AIDS, or any other malady that they may sometimes feel helpless or hopeless about. I do not represent any 12-step program other than HIV Anonymous. Though I have attended and continue to benefit from the teachings of other recovery programs, philosophies, religions, etc., I do not claim to be an example of how they work (or do not work). I can only speak for myself and tell you what has been my experience and has worked for me thus far. I have been blessed to survive many hard, lonely and confusing years of addictions, AIDS, and the trauma of growing up a Black man in America. I hope that you will identify with my story on some level, and will use it to help you to heal.

There are, in my opinion, many contributing factors to the mental, physical, emotional and spiritual state of being experienced in the world today. That is particularly true of Africans in America and worldwide. All of us are dealing with a form of posttraumatic stress. My personal journey has allowed me to still be alive, through God's grace.

I know what has worked for me, or at least I can recall some of the methods I have used to stay healthy. Many people ask me how it has been that there are so many people who have died with HIV/AIDS and yet I have survived so long. That is a question that I have had to ask myself many times. My first answer always has to be that it is the grace of God. Then I tell them about how attitude, nutrition and desire have played a part as well.

***

Joy is the freedom of expression without judgment, the freedom of being without fear or guilt. It is knowing that you are creating life on your own terms. It is the sublime movement of self allowed."— Ramtha

Any and all healing that I have experienced has been due to the Grace and mercy of my loving God and Creator. I can not stress this fact enough. I have had to learn how to accept and feel worthy of these blessings. I never want to lose sight of the fact that even though I have had to take certain steps in order to recover, it is my relationship with a God of my own understanding that is the most important thing to me.

In a touchingly loving naming ceremony, an African queen named Malaika gave my name to me. She chose the name Jelani Elekezana and when I asked the meaning of my name she told me the meaning was "worthy." I humbly accept these blessings, which include my name.

My life has been a series of miracles that have driven me, not allowing me to be at peace unless I wrote this book. It has been since 1988 that I have lived with the diagnosis of HIV. I had not had a drink or drug since 1985. I had, until 1985, been an IV drug user and had been having unprotected sex quite frequently. If you believe that IV drug use and unprotected sex are two of the more prevalent ways to contract the disease, then it is probably the way I contracted HIV in 1984. How I contracted the disease may not be as simple as that. It probably is not the most important thing. The fact that it marked a change in the way I perceived life is a more important point.

My drug addiction humbled me to the point of surrender. Admitting that I was powerless over drugs and alcohol and that my life had become unmanageable was a turning point in my life. It was then that I became teachable. That is when I was rescued from the grips of the insanity of using. The realization of the fact that I did not have to live any more than one day at a time was quite revolutionary and it freed me up to begin to learn who I was and work towards who I thought God wanted me to be. Thank goodness that is still what I am being.

Since January 29th, 1985, when I got clean from heroin, cocaine, marijuana, alcohol and whatever else I could get my hands on to make me feel better or at least different—until now—I have known many friends and family who have become casualties of this war. There have been too many to name, lest I forget to mention some. Many had already put their lives of using drugs and alcohol behind them. Most were finally experiencing the happy, joyous and free life without the shackles of active addiction. It is a sad irony that after years of living in the prison of our own minds, we would have to fight an even more lethal enemy. As slaves to our addictions, we were like soldiers on the front lines, bullets whizzing overhead. Every now and then, someone would take a bullet and die. Then, after getting clean and finding out that we had been infected with and affected by diseases like HIV, was like finding out that there was Agent Orange used on you by your allies in the battle. Fearfully, we knew that there would indeed be some "collateral damage." We had no way of knowing he extent of the carnage.

I say that as a way of dating my progression. After being asymptomatic for years, then developing full-blown AIDS, I was given only months to live. I continue to be blessed to be of sound mind and body. In my heart I feel I am now healed. I need to believe that in every cell of my body. There have been times when the virus has been undetectable in my blood while using medications and dormant even when I am not. There have also been times when my T-cell count has been as low as 2 (normal range is 650-1500) and I have had a very high viral load and been in the best of health. T-cells and viral loads are the way that the medical profession measures one's ability to fight off opportunistic diseases. My numbers often have not been what they consider to be good. I take their counsel, but I have learned not to live my life in fear of what could happen. That is not to say that I am not conscious of the possibilities, it just makes the experiment more real. It is a greater test of faith.

The effect of using medications has worked—whether it is important, and how important it is, is another story. I prefer not to use them but I thank God for the option. I know that the people that I last shared a syringe and cooker with on the streets of Jamaica, Queens, are all dead. There have been many times I wondered why I was still here and what it was that God is saving me for. Recently, while watching the adventures of my life unfold, I have had an epiphany. It may be as simple as living my truth and telling my story. It is because of this that I feel compelled to share my story with you. I do mean you specifically because there are no coincidences; and since you are reading this, it is somehow meant for you.

There are many people whom I know have been the voice and will of the Creator. In reality, we are all co-creators of our reality. I have had some wonderful teachers on this journey. Without their counsel and example, I would have been, well, I don't know where I would be. I do know that there are far too many people that I have known personally, that have succumbed to AIDS, alcoholism, drug addiction and other diseases. I had, until recently, shared with very few of them what my reality was in terms of having been diagnosed HIV positive myself. I don't know why, but I felt that by sharing how I was living and how I was integrating the wonderful life-saving information into my behavior would help them. I shared, with all that would listen, the power of participating in one's own survival.

That is not to say that they all gave up on life. I know that sometimes I feel like it would be easy to give up to the fears about death. Life has not been without challenges. I have had both conscious and unconscious bouts with depression. I am sure that many people get trapped in the prison of fear, guilt and shame.

I do believe that most of those who are now gone did not give themselves the best chance for survival by changing their lifestyle. It has caused me to understand the power of freedom. One of the greatest freedoms is from the slavery of my own desires. I am not seeking perfection. I am working for spiritual progress. The real blessing for me is that I have been exposed to information that, when implemented, has been of great assistance in that change in lifestyle. That has not only saved my life, it has improved my quality of life immensely. Having a program to live by has been great. From that I continue to learn. I pray for the strength to continue to practice the discipline I will need to give life my best shot, and to serve God more fully.

...surrendering is not giving up anything or becoming submissive to the world. We still have to live in the world. We can live in the world but not be of it. It is not the outer world that I am speaking of when I say that we are to surrender to heal. We still exist in the physical realm, and have to interact with other humans who may or may not be conscious of their actions or their own existence. We are not to be doormats. When we are able to remember to face fear and confusion with love, we change ourselves, those souls we interact with, and thereby we are changing the universe and shifting the paradigm.

Ekhart Tolle—"Power of Now"

THAT'S THE WAY OF THE WORLD

"...child is born with a heart of gold, way of the world, makes his heart so cold."—Earth, Wind & Fire

I was born and raised on the south side of Jamaica, Queens. It was October 11th, 1956, a time when Jackie Robinson, Y.A.Tittle and Sugar Ray Robinson were doin' their thing. It was when the skies were really blue, the air was still pretty fresh, and milk was delivered in bottles and would actually spoil after a few days in and out of the refrigerator. The neighborhoods were relatively crime free. People were still able to leave their doors open—compared to the more urban environments of Brooklyn, Bronx and Manhattan, Queens was basically considered prime farmland.

There were plenty of farms and trees in Queens, too. It was the home to the city's two horse racing venues and was bordered by the city's international airport, then called Idewild. The more heavily populated and urban boroughs of Brooklyn, Manhattan and the Bronx were the places that people escaping racism, farmlands, and unemployment of the South settled into first. The excitement of the city, with its bright lights, subways, tall buildings and fast pace was the antithesis of the tree-lined, slower paced existence in the southern states that most had escaped. Most came north to escape Jim Crow and to find work. The "city" was really very different from the vibe in

Queens. For those who felt that the transition from the south to New York was too drastic, Queens would provide safe haven as well as easy access to this cultural mecca.

Urban living held a great allure for those simple folk who had spent their earlier years dreaming of the chance to live in the greatest city on earth, New York. A large percentage of those who had migrated from places like Waterloo and Pineville, South Carolina would find some kind of social balance and evolutionary equilibrium in the slower and greener environments of either Queens or Long Island. Many of those souls who had been born and bred in a time and place where hard farm work was the norm, ended up in Queens. It seemed that with hard work and a dream, a person could do really well in New York. People from the south particularly liked Queens because it was the blend between the metropolitan, raucous city life and the industrious, home-owning, space-having country life that their DNA was more familiar with. The partying was good and accessible, but the transition from what it was like, to this new way of life, was less intense for some of those who needed more time to get used to it. We were living just enough for the city.

That is where my parents Leroy and Ethel Louise Smith, formerly Ethel Louise Middleton, both of South Carolina, had decided to settle down and raise a family. There was a great deal of partying that went on for them, as legend would have it. There are many stories of the revelry that they enjoyed both separately and together, with some of their life long friends. My mother had followed her older sister Leila to the north, coming up from Charleston, South Carolina. Aunt Leila had come north to Philadelphia years earlier. They did as many families did back then. They rode the Greyhound, or as it was said, they rode the dog up north and stayed with an aunt while working her way into independence. Though my mother had it pretty good living with her mother and step father, she decided at the age of 16 that she would prefer the bright city lights to the comfort of working in the country store that her step father owned near Meeting Street. So against her older sister's advice, she came north to find fortune and fun.

My father was a lot more motivated to get away from the country. He was getting away from the rigors of farm life, which surely were wearing him out. Roy, as he was affectionately known, would always tell the story that if a mule was sitting in his lap, he still would not tell him to giddyap. That was his way of saying how tired he was with having to plow the fields of his family's farm with a very stubborn mule. His grandparents reared my father in a small sleepy town called Waterloo, South Carolina. He lived there while his mother and sister made their way to Manhattan. It seems that my father had bit of resentment with his mother for leaving him on the farm so long, but that was not because she abandoned him. It probably seemed to her like the right thing to do. Maybe she had an idea about how the city would affect him. Time would tell the story more clearly.

It is always amazing the way that fate works to bring two people together, and then how they bring children into the world. That is the way of the world. A child is born with a heart of gold, then the way of the world makes his heart so cold. It is not that Roy and "Lou" came from such different worlds. It is just interesting to me how they came together. In their own individual ways, their lives were creating a desire for both of them to have children. Clearly they both wanted the kind of love that they felt they could cultivate from their own offspring. They both had experiences in their own lives that they wanted to make sure were not duplicated in the lives of their children. That conscious or unconscious thought is where I was conceived through them. The rest was merely a formality.

I distinctly remember two things that happened to my soul before I came back into this life. The first is that I drowned in my last life here on earth. My mind can recall that whatever entity my soul was living in, seemed to expire while gazing helplessly at the sun. At first there was a struggle to survive, and then a calm acceptance as I left that life beneath the ripples in the ocean. I have often romanticized that I was a captive on a slave ship that had just left Jamaica, West Indies when I was either thrown off the ship for being rebellious, or jumped off in protest of being held hostage. That would explain my love of Jamaica—and my need to be free.

The second event that I can recall is that when my soul was being placed into this being for incarnation, I was petitioning the Creator to not send me back here to this earthly plane. I can picture being cast out and traveling down a long tunnel, away from the light. It seemed like I was reluctantly descending through the birth canal. Though I had the feeling that I was voicing my displeasure for having to leave the peace and serenity of the place where "I" was dwelling, I did not actually yell until that damn doctor made me cry. He did not have to do that. I would have soon been crying plenty without any help.

On that eleventh day in October 1956, eight days after Roy's birthday, and years after Louise had silently petitioned the Creator for a manchild she could shower her love on, I, Reginald Leroy Smith, was born. It had to be then, under the Libra sun, and it had to be them to give me the best chances of learning the lessons of this life. Such is the case for us all.

I was born and raised on the south side of Jamaica,

Queens. It was a neighborhood full of contradictions, set on the edges of the racially segregationist views of Howard Beach, and just south of the economically bustling Jamaica Avenue, where all the surrounding neighborhoods shopped for their wares. If you walked a little ways to the south you would end up with your hat floating in the Long Island Sound. We were bordered by one of the most famous international airports in the world then called Idewild, now Kennedy airport. We lived next to St. Albans, where great musicians like James Brown, Count Basie and Duke Ellington had homes among the Black elite. Dichotomies abound: none were any more glaring than the contrast between the thriving communities that surrounded, and fed off, the constantly struggling south side of Jamaica, Queens (SSJQ). That is where the labor force that these communities, and the entire city, was fed from.

Like many, we were victims caught up in the so-called war on drugs, increasing crime and oppression of black folks in general. My family lived in a certain denial of the effects that society was having on our lives. Maybe it just seemed that way because I was a child somewhat shielded from some of the harsh realities of life. Living in denial was just that much easier to do back then because on the outside it seemed as if this was a normal environment. Indeed, it was very normal by the standards we were led to believe and expect.

Even at a very young age, I was deeply affected by injustice. My mother still does not believe that I remember some of the things that I do remember from when I was only months old. The first house that I lived in back in 1956 was on South Road, right in the heart of the south side of Jamaica Queens. It was an old two story brick colonial, hidden by oak and pine trees directly across the street from a Catholic Church and rectory. It had a bleached white brick and looked like a castle. The church buildings stood out amongst the other different types of architecture in the rest of the community.

I know that I was only months old when we lived there, but I distinctly remember being carried up the stairs to the second floor apartment that my parents were renting from Mrs. Aikens, whom I remember as a large, happy woman with an imposing black mole on her cheek. I remember the layout of the apartment with uncanny clarity. Mostly, I remember my father holding me in his hands, way above his head while lying on his back on the bed. He would toss me up and in return for the lovingly exciting ride, I would dribble and spit all over him and pull the hair on his face. Yeah, I know. Mostly any kid could probably say that they remember that kind of a scene. I really do. But then, I distinctly remember drowning in my last life and desperately petitioning our creator not to send me back to this earthly plane. Anyway, here we are.

It was not long before our family expanded and we would have to move. As a matter of fact, my sister, Pamela, was born some eleven months after me. You can do the math. With some help from my parents' very best friends, George and Deliah, we bought a two-story, single family house about a mile outside of the airport. It was a quiet neighborhood except for the sound of the jet planes that frequently seemed to be using our street to line up their landing approach. The planes were loud and flew close. The plane that actually crashed in the swamp six blocks from the house, across the street from our elementary school, accentuated that fact.

Our area was filled with middle class working folk who had migrated north in search of freedom and opportunity. There was still some racial diversity in the neighborhood. It would be a while before white folks were mostly all gone from this section of SSJQ. I know they hated to leave, but such was the nature of "white flight." When black folks moved in, they moved out. This was the late 50's early 60's. That was the way of the world.

***

The block on which I was to spend my most formative years was the epitome of normalcy, at least cosmetically. It was a tree-lined block of new homes built on a lot that used to separate the neighborhood in a most peculiar way. The houses in every direction that surrounded our block were much older. We did everything that a kid could want to do to have fun. Where we lived, there were some of the most intelligent and gifted kids that never got to live up to their potential. Many of us would never get to live the dream because we would become victims in one way or another. This was a war that we hardly had the chance to survive. The lengths to which our enemy, the ominous and nefarious "powers that be," would go to destroy us, were great.

There were four of us in the family. As I mentioned, my father and mother were hardworking products of South Carolina farm life. Though my mother was moved soon after her fourth birthday to more metropolitan Charleston, South Carolina, to live with her mother and step-father, they both knew what hard work was. Neither of them was opposed to doing what was needed to get ahead. My parents both possessed that same kind of work ethic that would be a life-saving example for me. Contrary to the popular perception that Black folks were lazy, my folks' attitudes about work were the norm, not the exception. Their generation seemed to know how to do both party and be responsible for the most part. The biggest demon they had to fight, besides racism, was alcohol. Alcohol was a monkey on their backs compared to the gorillas that the next generation, my generation, would have to wrestle with. The enemy would infiltrate our generation with all kinds of drugs for us to add to the alcohol. They did it in such a smooth way that we never even knew what hit us. We thought it was an escape route, but it ended up being the road to hell.

My sister and I were born eleven months apart, with me being the elder of us. It took me a while to realize why the fact that we were only eleven months apart was such a sly joke in family gatherings. I guess that six-week thing that doctors always tell new parents they should use as a rest period did not mean a damn thing to my father. I blame him because I know my saintly mother was an unwilling participant in that encounter. Not long after I was born, my mother quit her job at the telephone company to be able to spend more time at home with me (and with my father too, I guess). My father worked for the transit authority as a conductor on the trains. In the sixties, this was really good for black folks. He had a job with benefits. A good paying job and medical coverage was what we strived for. My father was a good provider for the family. We seemed to be living the American dream.

Everything seemed normal to me, including the neighborhood. We had a lot of fun growing up. We did everything you could do with a Pensy Pinky. That was the brand name of the little rubber ball that was the preference of our youth. The other balls were deemed to be mere imitations. We played stickball, handball, stoopball, aw man, those were some good old times. I was always really good at sports. When I got skipped from the second grade to the third at Easter time, it caused me to not only be a grade ahead, but two or three years behind my classmates age because my birthday is in October. My mother was able to get me into school when I was four years old because school started in September in New York. I never missed a beat with the fellas by being younger though, because I could hold my own in any sport.

They accepted me right away. It was the girls that seemed to be more mature and much more intimidating to me. Though we were all very young, and sex probably should not have been as much a factor in male-female relationships at that time, it certainly was on my mind. I guess I was a horny little boy. In Mrs. Ross' class in the second grade, my main man Tony and I used to giggle and laugh as we pulled the crotch of our pants taut so as to more clearly define and show each other our young "boners." We would intentionally let the girls "mistakenly" discover us doing this with the hope that it would interest them too.

I played Scrooge in the school play back in fourth grade. That was a good year. It was the starring role with twenty-six pages of dialogue. The objective of making me the star of the play was to keep me challenged and busy. I had already shown a propensity for bucking authority. I had the talent and intelligence to pull it off, though. It was a lot of work being an actor. I learned my lines and carried the role so well that I received rave reviews from the teachers, parents and, more importantly to me, my peers. Their teasing was good-natured and indicated their respect for the task I had accomplished. Little did I know that I would soon take on the emotions evoked by the angry Mr. Scrooge.

As a matter of fact, I guess the apple didn't fall to far away from the tree because it was in the fourth grade that I enjoyed my first adventures with sex. Yep, that's right. I don't know when my father had his first sexual encounter but I assumed that he was pretty fast. That is what the quick turnaround between my sister's birth and mine indicated. I certainly was a bit preoccupied with sex at a premature age. For most of the entire forth grade I would meet my little girlfriend Kay on the "back staircase" where we would proceed to engage in the kind of carnal education that made school worth going to. We would have our own little code so Mr. Granger, our rather large, dark-skinned teacher wouldn't know. It was the secret looks and the deception of all of our friends that made it so very, very exciting.

If some of my more popular and influential classmates or any of Kay's or my friends had known what we were doing, they surely would have busted up our daily tryst. One of her friends became suspicious of both of us secretly disappearing at the same time every day. That is how she found out after a year and a half of us keeping our secret, that Kay and I were finding ways to slip off to the back staircase. I did not know it then, but it was a lifetime friendship that we were developing and I felt pretty lucky to be sharing those kisses and warm embraces with someone like Kay. She may not have been considered the most "fine" little girl in the fourth grade, but that was because of her being dark skinned and having short hair. In the sixties, light-skinned people were in vogue. I really liked Kay, though, and thought she was really cute. She liked to play sports, had a wonderful smile, and she liked me. I could see the beauty in her.

Ultimately, her friend went out of her way to wait until Kay and I were at our spot, doing our thing, to sneak up and catch us. "Ooohhh, I am gonna tell!" is all I heard as Wanda giggled at her discovery. I don't know if I was embarrassed for having been caught, or relieved that someone else knew. After a year and a half, it was still fun and exciting, but I kind of wanted someone else to know how lucky I was. After that I got to spend the entire recess-playing ball in the schoolyard with my friends.

It felt good being "loved." My friendships like the one's with Kay and Tony were important to me. Though we were young and doing things that involved our natural adolescent sexual curiosity, the relationships meant much more than that. Our parents knew each other from the community. My mother was a beautician, so she did the hair of some of my classmates and their mothers. That being the case, I had a special—outside of school—relationship with some of the girls whose hair my mother did. Kay's mother and grandmother got their hair done at my mother's "shop." Seeing them with their hair wet or in curlers seemed to reinforce our friendships, once they got past the initial embarrassment. The way some of them looked when they came in made it evident that they would have to count on my discretion. I maintained their trust by never saying anything about it in mixed company. I was getting good at keeping secrets.

My mother had conveniently moved to work right around the corner from my elementary school. She did a lot of running back and forth to school to hear about my battles with school authority. For some reason I was an angry little boy, so having friends and playing sports were the ways that I coped with life. Maybe I was mad at God for sending me back to earth. I really don't know. That angry behavior is part of the reason why my mother and the teachers were creating ways to keep me busy and active. I was creating ways for myself to be happier. Hugging and kissing Kay secretly on the back staircase behind the auditorium was happiness to me.

It was not always easy for me to find a way to get away from our daily game of "punchball" at recess, but it was always worth the try. Being the youngest one of the guys, I still was always one of the first to be picked to play on a team. That was a honor in of itself. But Kay was letting me put my finger in a place where my instincts directed it and I thought that true love resided there. The sneaky adventure provided a behavior that would provide me with the chance to learn a life lesson. At least it was a recurring theme for me. There was a competition in my head for the time and effort that would go into both sexual gratification and satisfying my ego, or doing what would achieve greater self-awareness. It would surely be a pattern in my life and the choice has never been an easy one. I guess it is true what they say about those being our formative years.

Whether I was enjoying school prior to or after that was debatable. The reason I was skipped was because the administration and my parents were tired of me throwing tantrums, cursing out teachers and generally acting out. It seemed as if I had (and still have) a serious disdain for authority. Their answer to my disruptive behavior was to try to occupy me with more challenges. I was overachieving scholastically without any real effort, so I guess it made sense to consider moving me up a grade so I would have more challenging work and situations.

As shy as I was, and as angry as I was, I was surely happy to have been skipped. I already had friends in the next grade. If nothing else, I would be finished with school that much sooner. I liked the idea of graduating high school at the age of 16. I liked the idea of getting to the finish of this part of life sooner. Maybe being "grown" would allow me the ability to challenge authority more effectively. I could tell people how I felt with even more conviction. I was telling teachers at that tender age that they could kiss my ass because they were not my father! What I was really feeling was that adults were dismissing me because I was a kid. Teachers felt that they were right all of the time, and I could not see how that could be if they were human just like me. It took me a while to figure out that my parents were human too, but I did not try that kind of talk with them.

It was really hard to figure out what I was so angry at. I do know that my sister seemed to be very different from me. She was shy too, but she did not act as angry as I. Her biggest challenge seemed to be making sure that we remembered how tender-headed she was. She made it exceedingly clear how much it hurt her to have her hair combed or braided. Though I never thought that she was fat, Pam was what some called pleasingly plump. She was big boned, but not to the point where it really mattered at all. At least, her weight did not matter to me. My mother seemed to be keeping an eye on it, though. There was not much that my mother was not keeping an eye on when it pertained to her children. With all the stuff that I was getting into I was getting a great deal of attention, both good and bad. It was pretty clear to me that she did not appreciate living in the shadow of an older brother who appeared to be taking up more than his share of attention. Despite that, we forged a bond through all that we went through together. There was plenty of stuff going on between our parents at the house, and Pam and I were the only ones who really knew the extent of the drama.

With both of our parents working, Pam and I were often home alone. I guess that Pam kind of disliked authority in her own way, especially if it was coming from me. After all, I was not that much older than her and my sense of justice was weighted by my desire to not have to do the dishes or any other chore that would keep me from being able to do what I was obviously born to do—play. Anything that I could come up with to get her to do my chores was fair game. For a while it seemed necessary to make her believe that she was actually adopted and left on our stoop in a basket. That turned out to be rather effective and somewhat cruel. I was just playing with her. Who knew that she would possibly think it may be true? I thought she knew that she looked like our father and his side of the family.

That little tease seemed to reinforce her idea that I was being treated special by my parents because I was first. The idea of that planted the seeds of doubt in the way household justice was being handled by our parents. After all, I had been here first and had the advantage of having had eleven more months to work on them.

So, though we were so close in age, there were two grades between us after I was skipped. It meant that we would always be creating separate identities for ourselves. In her case, following in my footsteps would have been no bargain. I, on the other hand, would benefit from the pleasure of meeting more than one of her friends. For a horny little boy like me, that one benefit alone was worth plenty. I would benefit more than once from this arrangement. Between my mother being a beautician and having a younger sister so close in age, I seemed to be in pretty good shape as far as opportunities to meet girls was concerned.

My mother was the type to make sure that we both stayed very active. Scouts, sports, music, traveling—anything to keep us from getting caught up in the war being waged on the streets for our souls. Moms did whatever she could to make sure that our minds and bodies had something creative to do. It was no easy job for her to keep an eye on me. She had given up her job at the telephone company after I was born. It was a job she was very proud to have gotten and kept. It was a job that was the badge of accomplishment for a young lady who was the next to last child of five children. My mother had not graduated from high school, but had the courage to leave her home in Charleston, South Carolina at the age of sixteen to come north and live her dreams of city lights and party nights. I guess she, too, had a strong desire to be free.

I believe that there was some things going on in her step-father's house that caused her to want to flee. I am told that not long after my mother left home, her mother came north to live as well. I assume that there were some problems at the house. I know my mother had issues about the relationship between her mother and stepfather. What is not clear is whether or not my mother's strained relationship with her biological father had contributed to her discontent. Maybe all of the above played a part in the decision-making and character building process.

Whatever the case, Louise had developed the reputation for being a very conscientious parent. Though we are Black, and Black mothers loved their children just as much as any other race, there was some pride that my mother took in being considered a "Jewish mother" kind of personality. She has always wanted the best for her children and her family and she would go to any lengths to get it. Mom had to be strong because she was fighting what some may say was a losing battle. She had decided that "doing hair" would give her the independence and income that she would need in order to be the mother that she wanted to be, yet make enough money to maintain the independence she would need. Maintaining her identity in a marriage that had issues, and a society that worked against her, was a challenge. Most of the things that were going on in my world were still quite innocent at the time. In time that would surely change. After all, that's the way of the world.

WHEN DOVES CRY

....maybe I'm just too demanding, maybe I'm just
like my father—too bold.
Maybe I'm just like my mother, she's never satisfied.
Why can't they live with each other? This is what it
sounds like when doves cry.
Prince

My mother was quite at home with the group of
friends that she and my father had. The core group
of their friends was made up of three families. We
were all very close and all of us kids were pretty close in age,
so even when I could not be in the street I still had some
friends to hang with. Wayne, who was George and Delia's
son, and Curtis, Tracy and Marie's son, are my oldest friends.
I have known them all of my life and George and Delia are
like parents to me as well. They all were known to have had
a drink or two at any given time. My mother, though more
reserved than the others, certainly drank no less than they did.
They were just having some fun while dealing in a world that
did not have their welfare and upward mobility as a care or
concern. It never hurt anybody to have a drink or two, right?

I used to love the friendship and camaraderie they showed
each other. There is nothing that sticks out in my mind
more distinctly than waking up on Sunday mornings to the
sound of the six of them seemingly arguing in the kitchen.

The fact is that they were not arguing at all. They would be enthusiastically debating the topics of the day over bottles of a good bottle of Johnnie Walker Red or maybe some Chivas Regal. The Smirnoff Vodka was for my father's very best friend, my godfather George. Those were the days that I learned a great deal about creating an opinion, reading between the lines of bullshit, what friendship is and that Sunday breakfast is made of Grits and bacon.

Just because it was Sunday morning and most people were going to church was irrelevant. My mother would sometimes get us off to church. I guess now would be a good time to ask God's forgiveness for stealing the offering money she gave us and buying candy. I am sure God has a long line waiting of people confessing to that one. Most of the time though, we would just lie in bed and listen to the witty conversations, jokes and stories about "back in the day." The politics and opinions about whatever was happening in the world that week were what interested me the most. This was my real newscast, and I was getting it live and direct right there in my kitchen. This was a microcosm of what was going on in the world. Everyone in the world knew what was going on. Everyone knew that there was plenty of injustice in the world. Hell, it had not been too long since Black folks had taken some all-important steps in our struggle for self-determination and comparable opportunities. Rosa Parks had displayed the kind of courage that I saw in the women in my life display regularly. Her plight was representative of what we were enduring at the time.

The fact is that white people were suffering too, because they had to know that it would not be long before they would have to put their contingency plans in effect. Social consciousness was being raised. Organizations like the NAACP,

Black Panther Party, and The Nation of Islam were helping Black people identify themselves, and creating ways to change the way the system that had shackled the minds, hearts and aspirations of so many that had come before, and shift the ways that we would rebel. For white folks, that would mean things like COINTELPRO, terrorism by murder, and the biological annihilation with drugs, alcohol and disease. They would use some of these and more to maintain a sense of superiority over those in opposition to their twisted sense of entitlement. Well, some white folks anyway.

The point is that it made for an uncomfortable situation for the world. Racism pointed out so very clearly the hypocrisy of American democracy. On the one hand you had the traditional American call for freedom and justice for all, and on the other hand you had the blatant and indignant forms of racial discrimination right here in the great USA. Our parents' generation was very much aware of the past transgressions of the dominant culture. They were very suspicious of white people in general, and politicians in particular. They had begun to benefit from some of the changes that were being fought for. My parents and their generation were the catalyst for that change. They fought for social change for the benefit of their children, for the most part. They were intent on creating greater opportunity in the way they could best see a leveling of the playing field. There was so much that needed changing, but the education issue seemed to ignite great passions for those who felt it would afford Black people the opportunity to compete on an level field. Then again, there were many folks that would have rather died, at the time, than move away from their oppressive stance on equal rights.

For Black folks it meant having to choose whether you felt more comfortable with the peaceful, non-violent tactics of Rev.

Dr. Martin Luther King, or the more confrontational style of either the Black Panther Party or Brother Malcolm X. Would we follow the example of a sports legend and racial pioneer, Jackie Robinson, who with his quiet determination was changing people's ideas about our race? He did this with his workmanlike behavior and more docile attitude. There were many who felt more motivated towards action, and tended to follow the lead of the more gregarious and ostentatious Cassius Clay /Muhammad Ali. In different ways they all resonated with some sections of the black and white communities, one way or the other. Either way, the solution to the social "unrest" of the times was predictably enough dealt with in diabolical fashions. We could only guess and imagine the extent of the subterfuge that our own government would go to in order to quell what was being considered an internal threat and insurrection by "Negroes."

What the plan for pacification meant is that there would be lots of drugs and alcohol being placed in the Negro community for all the kids to have "fun" with. This is the way that the United States government decided it would make sure that it was able to maintain its control of the Black population in America, and affect the strength of its economic and political power for generations to come. Many would go to jail for crimes surrounding the getting, using and selling of drugs. They would become prisoners of war. Many would become political prisoners, especially those who would join and actively participate in the insurrection.

While young black men were being asked to give their lives to fight in wars overseas for the freedom of many other human beings, families in the SSJQ were suffering immeasurably from the decimation being caused by the suddenly heavy influx of heroin into the "inner cities" of America. Looming always was the possibility that your male friends or yourself would be "drafted" into armed service and forced to kill. When that happened, you would have to make the decision to serve or desert. That was not much of a choice.

It is no coincidence that heroin and alcohol, as well as methadone and other drugs, had such a deleterious effect on the entire community. The sight of grimy dope fiends running in and out of shooting galleries, people nodding and dribbling in the parks and streets, and the trauma and deaths of those who would become casualties of a war that had been declared on the black community—these things were an everyday occurrence. It created posttraumatic stress for the entire community. Once again, fear and death were being used to keep the masses in line. J. Edgar Hoover was a cross dresser, but that did not mean that his feminine side would dominate and balance out his apparent disdain for the black race. He could still find plenty of mean spirited energy to wiretap and intimidate any African-American or otherwise, with any influence with those in the community. Those who would voice too loudly their displeasure with this self-serving style of American justice needed to be silenced. My generation would have to navigate this freshly planted minefield with a map drawn from old reconnaissance data. The previous generations had seen their share of carnage, but this was a biological warfare that we had yet to experience with this much vengeance. It was not unlike the atomic bomb our government dropped on the Japanese. Many people were walking around in a zombie-like state of mind, suffering from the shock of the bomb that had hit us, and the fallout was so pervasive as to affect every living thing with its toxic aftermath. That poisonous cloud would prove to be as devastating as the bomb itself.

Our neighborhoods were flooded with heroin from the

poppy fields of Viet Nam and Columbia. Our brothers and sons and husbands were dying and if they came home, they were returning maimed, disfigured and disillusioned. The people in the black community maintained the hope and character that had sustained them through Jim Crow and segregation. When the soldiers, especially black soldiers, returned from the battlefields abroad, they faced another insidious and potentially deadly enemy waiting for them at home—dope.

These things and more were the topics that were being discussed by my parents and their good friends over Johnnie Walker, Smirnoff, grits and bacon, while they did the "slop" on the parquet kitchen floor. The fact is that the elders in my life were both socially conscious and opinionated. When James Brown created the politically powerful song entitled "Say it Loud, I'm Black and I'm Proud," it gave us something to dance to that really had black folks feeling good about themselves. I do not recall ever seeing that song rated on American Bandstand. There did not seem to be any contradictions in discussing the serious, sobering state of affairs over drinks, not at all. It all seemed really cool. That is until the party was over and the friends went home. That is when the acknowledgment of life's reality and the personal pain it was causing kicked in. That is when the relationship between my parents seemed to take on another dimension.

My father was fighting a battle within himself. Unfortunately, his family was both the beneficiary and victim of the conflict. He had to know in his mind he was of high intellect. That intellect only emboldened the demons that he could never seem to satisfy. Even though he was very much loved and admired by all those who knew him, you could somehow tell that he did not feel like he was reaching his fullest potential.

Then there was the mystery of his past and why his relationship with his mother was as tense and strained as it was. I cannot remember the time when I spent any more that a few hours (if at all) with my grandmother when she had not either had or was looking for a drink. She was a wonderfully candid person who would drop her opinion on you whether you wanted it or not. Grandma was loving and caring; you just had to have skin thick enough to withstand her verbal assault, or courage strong enough to allow you penetrate her protective shield and seemingly unlimited arsenal of wit. It seemed sure Dad had some anger about his relationship with his mother, too. I later found out that it had something to do with Grandma leaving Dad on the farm in Laurens, South Carolina while she moved north with my aunt Vera. It was very evident that dad was harboring anger and resentment in the way he fought the most destructive of wars—the one he waged with my mother. I have no idea what went on in the relationships of the elders prior to my birth. They would talk about the good times, and sometimes about the bad, but the way they spoke of the past was usually in a general way. Family secrets were formed and maintained. Cracking that code would take more than a drink or two.

***

By the time I was in junior high school, Dad had taken a job on the police force. I am sure that he was drinking liquor long before he took that job, but there is no doubt that the job intensified his drinking. Now he was a man that was fighting many battles in this conflicted society. Besides whatever personal demons he may have been dealing with, he now went to work daily in the housing projects of New York City with the daily charge of finding ways to "keep the peace." At the very least, he would have to stay alive, get paid and take care of his family as best he could. He was a good provider for the family even if he sometimes had to be very creative about how he would provide a good life for us. He had done other jobs and probably could have been good at many more. Dad had a keen intellect and had inherited his wit and candor from his mother.

For a man like my father, with an innate sense of justice and humor, it still was hard to balance his job with the systemically oppressive and racially prejudiced justice system. His job was to find a way to use the law to serve and protect. Being a Black cop meant that you had to survive the animosity of some of his "sick white brothers," but he also had to police a war zone. Dad put his life on the line everyday because he believed that he had the charm and authority to help keep the peace. Everyday he worked in the ghettos in the most volatile environments in America—or the world for that matter. He was a housing cop in some of the most dangerous housing projects in Brooklyn and Manhattan. You would think that the respect that Dad gained from his constituents by successfully negotiating these demilitarized zones would be satisfying to him.

You would think it might be satisfying enough, and possibly make him eligible for a medal. Instead, he had to fight to maintain his dignity in a society that seemed intent on depriving him of it. Somehow, he needed to use the law to protect those who needed to be protected from those of us who would be victims turned predators. That was a complication that seemed to find some relief in "the bottle."

***

There were many wars going on in our neighborhood. The contrast between what was going on "out there" in the world, like the Civil Rights Movement and the Cuban Missile crisis, and what was going on in our home and family were strikingly similar. There were some conflicts going on in our own home that were hard to understand or believe. It was not what it appeared to be on the outside. Roy and Lou, like many other married couples, were withstanding the barrage of challenges caused by external pressures. Their relationship, like Cuba, was sure to be blown up if things did not change. That is just how like was life in America in those days. That is what life was like in my home and the homes of many living in the SSJQ.

My parents' war was the most impressionable. The things going on in the world at the time affected me. I was affected very deeply. The things going on up close and personal in my home affected me even more. We had a great neighborhood block to grow up on. The fact that we actually did live in a "ghetto" meant that you could expect all of the things that come along with Ghetto life. This is because of all the crime that was going on in the neighborhood. Most of the crimes were due in some way to the drugs flooding onto our streets. Prior to that you could still find many families keeping their doors unlocked or open all night. This was the beginning of social insecurity, the really new deal. It was probably no more crime than you would find in any other neighborhood. Somehow when it was portrayed in the media on the 6 & 11 o'clock news, all crime looked like Negroes were perpetrating it. I guess that scared everybody, even the majority of decent, hard working black folks living in our community.

The flashing lights from the police cars, ambulances and fire engines were the wallpaper that colored the walls of my room at night. The sirens were the lullabies that rocked me to sleep. Maybe it seemed like a scene right out of the movies. It seems like exaggeration that moviemakers make. When you live there you end up taking it for granted because you see it every day. Living inside the ghetto, we hardly even noticed the way it looks. For those who are not from the "ghetto" it must look different both live and in the movies.

The way that my parents would interact after their friends went home was different. Sometimes conversations and topical discussions would get tense while their friends were there, signaling the time for the party to break up. Somehow there would often be a point where too much liquor was imbibed and something was said that would cause my mother and father to argue. There were times when those arguments took a dramatic turn for the worse. Sometimes, my sister and I were left to make some life and death decisions—like if and when to call the police to break up the fighting. That was very embarrassing to do and it was against my better judgment to ever call on "the man" to handle anything.

We grew up only blocks from Yuseef Hawkins, a young man killed "mistakenly" by the police. I had heard of many others who had called the police to help solve a domestic dispute or otherwise only to become victims of "mistakes." Some had been shot by police officers multiple times—by mistake. If it happened around the corner from where we lived, it could surely happen here too.

Except for the fact that my father was a policeman himself, I would never have made that call. Their fraternity of policeman always afforded him the ability to escape arrest, and my sister and I just wanted the fighting to stop. So we made the call more often than we wanted. The police would come and make him leave. More times than not, that was all he wanted to do, anyway. When Dad started drinking, he usually did not stop until he got wherever it was he wanted to be. That was often somewhere between good times and oblivion. Many times that would be somewhere other than at home. Pops was well known in more than one of the neighborhood watering holes.

Such was the world of duality that we lived in. I had gratitude for having enough material things and friends to make life seem palatable. Yet I was surrounded by that kind of pain that showed up in lots of ways. I know that caused both embarrassment and the lies that tried to hide it. Undeniably it contributed to the way I would live. I never wanted to pick sides between them. I did not want to have to deal with trying to keep our family business out of the street. It wasn't like the neighbors did not know what was going on. Kids can surely be cruel enough to at least ask the question—what was going on at your house, man? I was ashamed to say. It was then that I guess I began to develop a plan on how I was going to negotiate my feelings in this world. I had already unconsciously begun to set up defense mechanisms that would soon just be "isms." I was beginning to add fuel to the fire that was being fanned by the winds of shame and guilt. Those "isms" would remain hidden from the world by my ego and image for years to come. You just can't keep that kind of thing silent for long. Sooner or later we all would have to pay the price.

THE WORLD IS A GHETTO

Don't you know that it's true, that for me and for you
the world is a ghetto?
War

Sure, there were drug dealers hanging out and making
deals on the corner. Yes, there were times when gunfire
punctuated the night air with the reminder that no
matter how "normal" our neighborhood looked, with its tree
lined streets and two family homes, we were still in a war
zone. When I think of the way that the media portrays what
a ghetto is supposed to look like, I get confused. I find it hard
to think of my block or neighborhood as a ghetto. There were
indeed some areas that were dilapidated and very poor. Our
block happened to not be one of those. On Inwood Street, the
lawns were manicured and the houses were well kept. That was
the case for most of the houses in the entire neighborhood. Life
was a lot rougher in the "projects." With people living on top
of each other in low-income housing, there was sure to be an
adventure. When you are living in the ghetto, you may realize
that there are certain things you may have to do to survive, but
you may not think of it as ghetto life. I guess that is some kind
of defense mechanism.

Maybe "ghetto" is a state of mind. Maybe it has nothing to
do with the mean income average for a particular community.
Is it possible that life was becoming a media fulfilling

prophecy? Which came first, the news or the anticipation of the news? Statistics said that there were more single white females on welfare than any other demographic, but every news story about that or any violent crime usually had some black person being hunted and/or feared. Dope was changing the neighborhood too much. People were becoming less likely to talk to each other. The pressure of life in the big city was starting to get to everyone. Most of the white folks had split and headed to the "suburbs." Whatever white folks that were left in the hood were either living this lifestyle with us by choice, or just caught up in the net with the rest of us fish. White folks that lived in the ghetto were either very happy to be able to get more than the regular white person's helping of "soul", or very angry for not getting the benefits of being white in a society that greatly benefited those who were white. Ghetto, though it may look Black on American television and movies, is about more than race or money. Ghetto is a state of mind.

There were many of my friends that lived in the neighborhood that were already dealing heroin, methadone and other hard drugs. On average there were plenty of 13 and 14 year olds that were sniffing dope, shooting dope and drinking wine. The illusion of hardworking two parent households belied the truth about what was going on in just about every home on the block that had children living in it, and that means almost all of the homes on the block. Somewhere along the line we had gone from playing stickball in the schoolyard of P.S. 123 to playing craps with the dice from the Monopoly game.

The enemy had slipped into our camp so quietly that we had gone from running relay races around the streets adjacent to Inwood Street, to running ourselves ragged making trips uptown to 116th Street in Harlem to buy heroin for our still adventurously amateur consumption. Most of them still seemed to be getting high because they wanted to, not because they had a habit. That would not last very long. How can you win when you are using heroin? When you start getting high to escape reality at such a young age, you never get to grow emotionally. When we started getting high, our emotional growth stopped.

At least some of us were still holding on to our amateur status. Some of the older guys, and not much older at that, had already figured out that they could make some money selling drugs in the neighborhood. Not only could they have the things that we were made to think were important to us, but they could be high and not have to worry about competing with the rest of the world for the jobs, careers and other material things our parents were working so hard for.

Those things, like cars, money, clothes and stuff, seemed somehow either out of the reach of those whose parents did not have it, or like something that was taken for granted by those of us who did. Most of us had not made up our minds about how we would get the finer things in life yet and were sure that we had plenty of time before we would have to decide on what kind of good job with benefits we would pursue. When it became important to figure it all out, we would surely find a way to get those things, because society dictated that we got them. That is what a successful person did, and we all planned on being successful. If selling and using drugs was the quickest and most feasible way to have the nicer things in life, like cars, money and the like, then many of us would ultimately be willing to take a shot at it. Many would get shot at in the process, just like on TV and in the movies. Now we were beginning to live the way we were being portrayed in the media. Life was imitating art.

Selling and using drugs was always an option. Heroin and marijuana were cheap, high quality and easy enough to get. Superfly was just one of the super cool, got it goin' on, I wanna be rich too, kind of images we were seeing in the movies and on TV. I don't know which was larger than life—the movies or reality. Guys my age were already getting busted and going to jail for having and selling drugs. Some were already their own best customers and getting high on their own supply.

Either way seemed to be just fine with most of white America. Most of those white politicians close enough to participate in change were caught up in the politics of the war being waged on the black community. I am sure that their strings were being pulled. That is how the game is played. My generation seemed less likely to be pacifist. My generation was rebellious. We had grown up in the times of great conflict and confrontation. We protested against the government because it was perpetuating the same kind of madness on the rest of the world that we, and our ancestors, had experienced first-hand. We knew that it was not right and we were willing to fight back much harder than our ancestors were able to. *Smiling faces, smiling faces tell lies, ain't it the truth. Smiling faces, smiling faces and I got proof...*

Our communities seemed to be growing poppy plants. How else could heroin be getting into our homes, noses and veins with increasing regularity? With the war in Viet Nam being fought at the same time you would think that the brothers coming home were bringing it back. That could not have been the case, because most of the brothers that made it back did so in a body bag.

I, for one, had not yet crossed that particular bridge. I had not yet started using drugs at all. Sure I had had the requisite amount of wine and knew what a buzz was. I had even gotten drunk one time while away at summer camp. It was the perfect opportunity for me to drink and get away with it, and it was the perfect reason for me to do so—to enjoy a party and be able to talk to a girl that I really liked but did not have the courage to talk to. Besides, at sleep away camp, I was safe away from the always-curious supervision of my mother. Even then I got so drunk that I spent what seemed like only five, maybe ten minutes at the party before I had to be carried back to my cabin. I woke up the next morning remembering little of what had transpired and having the most colossal hangover I had ever had. If this was the outcome of a night of drinking, I surely did not see what my father, with his many drunken episodes, and all of the rest of the guys nodding and throwing up from the effects of heroin, saw as the benefit.

I was still optimistic that my talent as an athlete might possibly provide me a way out. I most certainly had the talent and God given ability to achieve whatever I chose to pursue. Athletes were emerging as the new role models. That seemed to be the way to possibly make lots of money and live all my dreams. I had been blessed with certain athletic gifts that would give me hope of becoming a professional. I never really had the confidence to go after the dream.

One thing proved to be true. The more time we spent living in the environment, the greater the chance that the drugs, alcohol and jails would usurp mostly any ambition that would try to grow in the ghetto.

My father had this strange relationship with alcohol. I promised myself I would never grow up to be like him in that regard. That created quite a conflict in me. I loved and admired my father and aspired to be like him. He was an extremely witty and intelligent man. I hoped that he would pass that on to me. The fact is that I was already blessed with a fine, sharp mind and athletic body. I had a unique talent for jumping. I was gifted in that I could jump really high, a skill very handy especially when playing basketball. I would not have been the first to play their way out of the ghetto, but I lacked the confidence or work ethic that would make that dream of playing professional sports a reality for me.

That dream still held some allure for me when I decided to start hanging somewhere other than on the block that I lived. It was natural progression for a young man like myself to branch out and start to broaden the parameters of his world. Besides, I really needed to get away from all of the drama at the house. When I got a Neighborhood Youth Corps summer job at 14 years old, it was the beginning of the experience of independence. That would serve to be as much an aphrodisiac as any drug I have ever had. The timing was good for me to begin to be somewhere other than around my house. There was more drama going on there than I wanted to confront—or be reminded of by my not so diplomatic, sometimes cruel friends.

By the time I was in junior high, most of my friends and relatives were already very involved with drugs and alcohol. My friends had already been through drug "boot camp." Most were smoking pot and drinking wine and a good deal of them were sniffing and even mainlining heroin. In the most industrialized country in the world, (we are talking late '60s, early '70s) drugs and alcohol were rampant in my neighborhood. That could not have been by mistake. Still, I was looking for a way to escape the madness, one way or the other.

Even though our block was considered to be like an oasis in the desert, I could walk outside and go to the corner store and get any kind of drug that I wanted. If I went a couple of blocks either way, I would have to pass either a liquor store or bar before I could even get to the bus stop. There was always ample time to make the decision to buy a beer or pint of wine while waiting for the bus to come. The wait for the bus was usually long enough to go back and forth on whether to drink or not. Then I would have to choose to go to school or not. It was a decision made more than once.

If it were hot a cold beer would go down really nice. If it were cold, a half-pint of blackberry brandy would warm the cockles of my heart. It may get me through the day. It may change my day completely. Many a day has been changed for the worse while standing on Sutphin Boulevard waiting for the Q-6 bus to finally come.

The houses and the neighborhood were older once you got off my block of Inwood Street. That is not to say that the character of the people living on our block was any better than that of those good, hard-working folks that lived in the rest of the community. It just made it easier to have that kind of "across the tracks" mentality. It was not like we wore it on our sleeves, or even acknowledged it existed, but our street was made up of newer houses than most of the rest of the neighborhood.

Things did get a little rougher as you made your way across Sutphin Boulevard. Among other things, that is where all of the projects were. "Forty" Projects and Baisley Projects were a couple of projects that fit the description of "rougher." Life was different there. I think people there were just a little more desperate to find a way out of the battle because the situation was more intense. That was especially true of the folks living in "Forty" Projects. There were people living in the projects that had been battle tested and certainly seemed scarred from the experience. Once I left the block to explore my freedom to move around and see the world, I did not have to go far to be tested or tempted.

Being bussed to Junior High School way out in Floral Park with the white kids was supposed to be a privilege. It did not seem like it was going to work to my favor even if the schools were supposed to be better. It didn't seem like a blessing to have to get up 2 hours before the white kids who lived close by the school. Then, we would be expected to compete with those kids. We were also rising to the challenge of changing the racially biased mindset of all the generations that preceded us.

Even the name of the area surrounding the school sounded different. Floral Park sounded like they thought their shit didn't stink. In my heart I was very glad to not have to go to the school all of the other kids on the block were going to. From the horror stories I had heard from the kids one grade above us that lived on the block, going to Shimer Junior High was more of a gladiator school than anything else. In my heart of hearts, I still felt like a punk. I did not know for sure how much heart I had. I know I did not want to have to fight my way through school. That seemed a distinct possibility for those attending Shimer. Thank God—I was going to be bussed to the white school. Integration had its good points—kind of.

WE SHALL OVERCOME

We shall overcome, we shall over come, we shall over someday. Deep in my heart, I do believe, we shall overcome someday.
Rev. Dr. Martin Luther King, Jr.

I am sure that my mother had something to do with me going to JHS 172. She had a way of going out of her way to protect me. When you are young black man trying to hold his own in the ghetto, that kind of protection has its ups and downs. You can't claim that kind of protection outright without losing face. Like we used to say, you can't save your face and your ass at the same time. I admit that I am glad that she went out of her way to save my butt.

I loved my mother and respected her and her courage. She was the wife of a black cop who liked to drink. Sometimes when my father would be drinking, my mother and he would fuss and fight. It took a lot for her to deal with the pressure of that reality. No matter what was going on at home, my mother always had the time and energy to keep us involved in some kind of activity. She innately knew that would be one of the best ways to keep us out of trouble. For a long time, my mother's plan would work. I attended the YMCA, Boy Scouts, little league baseball and soon I would be playing organized basketball. I was able to get involved in whatever I was interested in. My mother drove my friends and me to many a little league baseball or basketball game.

By the time I started junior high school, my relationship with my mother had become somewhat strained. It seemed to me that whenever I was crazy enough to be honest with her about what I was feeling, it would somehow get turned around and used against me. I mean, my mother meant no harm, I know. I really wanted to prove my independence from my parents and everyone else. I guess that was regular for that age.

I made up my mind to never be complicit in my own demise. In other words, I was not going to give my mother, or anyone else, the emotional ammunition to use against me. So I learned how to hide all of the buttons to the control panel of my emotions. Consciously and unconsciously, I learned how to hide my feelings. I had been a crybaby in elementary school. Showing my feelings by crying was not winning me any cool points. I did not want to have to deal with that kind of ridicule all of my life so, I would have to stop all of that feeling stuff. That meant learning how to bottle my emotions.

I learned to hide my feelings long before I ever learned how to identify those feelings. Pain and fear were two of the feelings I knew and was trying to avoid. Those are the same feelings that would later in life come to eat me up. I guess the fruit doesn't fall too far from the tree. That seemed to be the same thing that my father was going through. Pain looked a lot different on him than it felt in me.

In the '60s and '70s, schools were just starting to be integrated. Most of the kids that lived on my block had been placed in Shimer Junior High School. Almost all of those kids who had been living on Inwood Street long enough had gone to the elementary school P.S.123, which was right on the next corner of Inwood Street, right across Foch Boulevard. Naturally, when most kids went into Junior High School, they went to the school in the neighborhood—Edgar D. Shimer High School. Who the hell is Edgar D. Shimer, anyway?

Nobody ever asked who Shimer was. That was not the most important question for those attending this school for budding gangsters and heroes. A much more prevailing thought on a daily basis was whether or not you were going to be able to keep your lunch money, sneakers, leather coat or anything else that someone else found to have value. Chances are you would have to fight one of the many more experienced and established predators in and around the school.

They had guys, and girls, so tough at that school that they would take your stuff for the fun of it. Fighting for your stuff was a sport at Shimer. I was not a fighter at that point. So, I breathed a sigh of relief when I found out that I would be taking the long, two-bus ride to the outskirts of Queens. At least there I would have a chance.

There was plenty of time on the bus rides to and from school to get into trouble. I had managed thus far to evade the mild amount of peer pressure that was being applied regarding getting high on drugs. Up to this point of my life I was still pretty innocent. I had not started getting high yet. One habit that I did start back then was smoking cigarettes. It was before they were known to be the killers that they are and at a time when it was definitely more cool to be smoking. If there was any peer pressure that I fell victim to, it was smoking out of the desire to be cool.

Being cool was no small chore. I already had to keep quiet about being so much younger than everyone else in my grade. If I could keep that secret well enough, I would not lose all of the cool points that came with being an athlete and having friends. There was no one else from Inwood Street that went to JHS 172 Queens. They all had to take their chances at Shimer.

But there were plenty of guys from the neighborhood that were a part of the bussing experiment like me. My "god brother/cousin" Wayne, whom I had known all my life, was one of the guys who went to school with me, and I was glad about that. At least there would be someone I really knew there with me. A lot of the guys I had gone to P.S. 45 would be going there with us as well.

It did not take long for me to make friends, though. Wayne was a year and a half older than I. He seemed much more experienced about girls and many other things. I am sure he was invited to way more hooky parties than I was, and of all the guys in junior high school, he ended up having the prettiest girlfriend. My claim to fame would be that my two best friends in junior high had the same last name as I. We came to be known as the Smith brothers. Nathan, David and I looked as different as we possibly could, so there was no mistaking us for blood brothers. Nathan looked Puerto Rican because of his fair skin and slick, jet-black hair. David was short and wore black framed glasses, and I was taller, like Nathan, but not as "yella." We did have lots of things in common, not the least of which was that none of us had a girlfriend. We all learned to smoke cigarettes together and we hung out at recess. Something else we had in common was that we did not participate in any of the race riots. Being among the first to racially integrate the entire New York City school system was challenging for all of us. The school we were now in was entirely white until we showed up. Those white kids, just like us black kids, were operating in part with information that had been given to us from a number of sources. Our parents, history, and the world at large were showing us how hard it was for the races to mix and coexist. Integration was the solution to the major disparity in education opportunity afforded to black kids. White folks had nice stuff and we wanted some of it. In the process we would sometimes "have misunderstandings". Because of that there were plenty of those race riots to avoid.

It was a two-fare zone and a two-bus ride daily trek to get to school. We would have been effectively "redlined" and deprived of attending the more respected suburban schools if we would have had to pay full fare to get back and forth. We got to see a lot more of Queens than I had previously seen, every day going to and from school. Being the kids we were, there were plenty of opportunities to get in trouble. Acting up on the bus, stealing candy from the corner store and smoking cigarettes were regular activities. We were lucky that we did not get caught or get into any serious trouble for the things that were said and done. We were not bad kids at all, just kids who innately knew that we were as good, or bad, as anyone else.

For the most part, Black and white kids in my world got along with each other rather nicely. It did not have to go down like that, though. I had seen the black kids and their parents in Alabama. They had to deal with an obstinate George Wallace and go head to head with the people of Birmingham for the right to do what we were getting ready to do. It did not register that we could be met at the school door with the same kind of opposition. After all, those were the "crackers" from the Deep South. It was like they were from another planet that seemed like it was many light years away.

This was the north. I knew that there was racism and injustice everywhere. It just never registered that it would be happening where I was. As it turns out, I am not sure which form of racism had more of an effect on me. The blatant, "we don't want you niggers around here," in your face kind of racism, or those whose attitude seemed to be that "you can send your kids to our schools and we won't say we don't want them here—but when school is over make sure they do not let sundown find them on this side of town." It was an attitude we had already seen in white neighborhoods much closer to home than Floral Park.

The same kind of fear mentality was enforced in Howard Beach. Howard Beach was a predominantly Italian neighborhood situated just down the road and across the Van Wyck and Belt Parkways. Black people were not allowed in the neighborhood at night and were barely tolerated in the daylight. You could catch a mob beat down in that part of town if the shade of your skin was brown. It is where reputed Mafia families lived and operated. The news archives are filled with incidents that were race related whether they are documented as such or not. There are even more stories of intimidation that will never be recorded.

That is the way that kind of racism showed up. They told us they just wanted to keep their neighborhoods safe. There was always the threat of violence. The attitude was that if black folks were allowed to just hang out in their neighborhoods, it would not be safe. I could not understand why it was that way, either. We were all supposed to be free, living in a free world. Why did white folks not like us Black folk?

Something was not right about the stuff they were teaching us in school. I mean, it made sense that if the Indians were already here in North America when Columbus got here, the Indians had to have discovered America, right? So what was all this about Columbus? The system and the things that we were taught in school was suspect to say the least. In its most devious form, this indoctrination was part of the conspiracy to govern by fear and deceit. If Thanksgiving really was when the settlers ripped off the Indians, then how come all the history books, movies and teachers made it seem like the white folks were the generous good guys? And this Boston Tea Party they had was about freedom from their British oppressors? There were obvious, and not so obvious, contradictions about the information we were getting taught in our schools.

Somebody was lying, and they had been lying for a really long time. The lies had gone on so long that a person was a radical if you attempted to question and expose this hypocrisy. Even as a child in elementary school I would get in trouble for questioning and challenging authority. The main reason I would act out and curse is because I felt disrespected and dismissed by adults simply because I was a child. My soul felt like it was older and wiser than my years. I knew something did not add up and I was smart enough to ask the question and be persistent enough to press for a believable answer. Not that authoritative "because I said so," either. That type of response would never do. I generally was very respectful, but I always had a "you ain't my father" kind of attitude. I would later in life understand more clearly that it was more of a "you ain't my Father God" attitude.

The fear and lies were part of what caused racism. They were part of why people did not want Black folks to sit with them on the bus, or eat with them at the lunch counter. How else could you explain that after having been raised and nurtured by our mothers, these same people who had been the nanny or housekeepers in their families for many years priornow acted like they were born into superiority by virtue of the color of their skin. How could you explain the hatred of some of our sick white brothers for Martin Luther King, Muhammad Ali and Malcolm X? We were all being lied to and white folks had reason to want to believe it. They were afraid there wasn't enough stuff to go around and that Black folk were going to use up more than "our share" of the stuff. Lord knows how little stuff that must have been, but in those white folks' estimation, it must have been more than they were willing to part with even if black folks had created and maintained most of the wealth America is so proud of

Black folks contributed to the way it was. We seemed intent on getting "our share" one way or the other. If there truly was a finite amount of stuff, and white folks had stolen it or had it built on the backs of others, then it made sense that black folks were trying to "get theirs" and white folks were trying to keep it. The way it looked to everybody on TV and in the movies is that black folks would beg, borrow or steal to get ahead. We believed that just like we went for the Columbus discovered America story.

So we rode the bus to school. We went because white folks had nice stuff. We went to get a "better" education and to have the opportunities that our parents did not get. The transition was somewhat painful. It seemed that the responsibility of the protecting the reputation of our entire race was in our adolescent hands. It was an unspoken pain. Not the kind of nationally televised pain of rock throwing, epitaph spitting "crackers" hating "niggers." It was the quiet acknowledgment that the world was an unfair place where people sometimes imposed injustice on each other and on everything else on the planet. I made up my mind back then that before I would accept the world like it was, I would die. I remember Moms always trying to tell me "That is the way the world is. You're just going to have to learn how to deal with it." I remember always thinking to myself that I wanted to be a part of changing the world. How was I going to change the world if I just accepted as it was, I thought.

There was some wisdom to what Moms was talking

about, though. I would have to learn how to either accept, or at least how to negotiate in the mine-filled battlefield of this world. We went to school in white neighborhoods and I got plenty of opportunities to learn new things about how to negotiate the world that was. There was more than one time when we had to leave school early and fast in order to get out of the area because of fights between the races. It seemed entirely too easy for a couple of carloads of white teenagers with chains to be chasing black students out of their area.

I am glad to say that even though I knew what was going on around me, and despised the fact that it was, I was able to get along with everyone, no matter what the persons' color or religion. I knew that the world in general could use some help in learning how to live in harmony, but I tried to get along with all the people in my world, no matter what color.

***

I had more problems with the white administration than with any other students. The teachers were more entrenched in their smug authoritative behavior. They had been raised in a different time and place. We clashed because, in my mind, I was stuck between a rock and a hard place. I did not like those teachers because they were being assholes, not because they were white. I had my battles with the black teachers, too.

It was an important part of my development as a person to learn how to deal with people of all races, especially white people. It was also an important part of our generation's history that we would a part of changing America and the world. Having lived this life at that particular time is a part of what makes me who I am. It added to my survival skills. It helped me to be able to navigate deeper into the jungle and endure. Later on in my life—and not that much later—I would have to use those skills to get by.

JOY AND PAIN

...are like sunshine and rain; they're both one in the same.
Frankie Beverly & Maze

A round the neighborhood, I had begun to make a name for myself as one of the better baseball players in our little league. Jamaica Central Little League was at the center of our lives back then. The older guys had moved on to the Pony leagues and we played Little League until we were 13. We took our baseball very seriously and there was so much talent in the league it was hard to stand out. Many of the best players in the league came from Inwood Street, the block that we lived on. The way we played ball everyday, it was no surprise that we would be as good at it as we were.

The parade that the league would have every year was the only parade in this part town. On the South Side of Jamaica Queens, there was no circus, parade or any other kind of fanfare. This yearly community ritual of an opening day parade for the young ballplayers, coaches, umpires and sponsors that made up Jamaica Central Little League, was a big deal for us. We really loved the excitement of getting our uniforms and season schedule a few days before the parade. We all would go the extra mile and press our uniforms, sometime with really well defined creases, and some spit shined cleats. We wanted to look especially good in the parade. If you were one of the lucky teams, you would get to play in front of what would probably be the largest crowd that we would see during the entire season. I sure got butterflies in my stomach on opening day.

By that time we would know which of our friends' teams we would play, and when. We would then proceed to sell the appropriate amount of wolf tickets to those who needed them. Things like our little league opening day parade were things we took a lot of pride in. For the kids it meant that we were valued by our elders and peers, and for the adults it was validation of their desire and ability to care and provide for their children. Sure, on any given day if you were to walk down Sutphin Boulevard you could expect to see lots of caring adults, or hear the blaring sirens emanating from either the fire engines or the police cars rushing along this major artery to another crisis situation. That still was going on opening day, but it was all put on hold while we did our thing .

The parade ran right down Sutphin Boulevard, in the center of the community. Parents, friends, store owners and the like, would all come out to support us. It was a big deal for days before, to get our uniforms ready for the parade. It was before we started our season, so the uniforms were still somewhat clean, as clean as they would be all season if you were playing. All of the kids from our block were starting on one team or the other. The uniforms were did wear were most likely handed down from the previous year's team. It was rare that we would get sponsored for new ones every year, though it did happen occasionally. We had some community business owners who sponsored teams in our league. Between the coaches, parents and sponsors, we were taken good care of. Whether the uniforms were new or not, we would spend time washing and pressing them to look good in the parade.

If your team would play a game on that day, it was like

being in the big leagues, and we made as much of it. During the season we kept our batting statistics for the season and could tell you at any given time what our batting average was from game to game. There were guys who did not do well in math in school, who could figure the earned run average of a pitcher or their own batting average in the blink of an eye.

The coaches and umpires that ran the league were real role models for us. The fact that they would take the time to pick us up, take us to practices and games, definitely kept us out of trouble. Playing for Mr. Harris who coached my team, the Phillies, and Mr. Holly, who coached our all-star team with him, was a real joy and a privilege. They taught us determination and helped us understand the importance of a good work ethic. They taught us even more by caring and consistently being there for a large number of kids. They deserve a lot of credit for what they did for us.

Mr. Riley and Mr. Jamison were our neighbors. Mr. Jamison lived next door and Mr. Riley lived down the street. They were the pony league coaches of my team, the Mets. That was so appropriate because I was a huge New York Met fan. The real professional Mets did not have ballplayers who were a whole lot better than us at the time. It was fun playing for them and it was easy to get a ride to practice and games. We could walk to any field that we had to play on, but we rarely had to.

It was fun watching Mr. Brooks with his flamboyant style of umpiring. He was very boisterous and demonstrative in the way he would call balls and strikes. Mr. Brooks had a distinctive umpiring style that we would always mimic. These black men were mentors and they provided many others with some of our fondest memories of our youth. It certainly bought me a few more years of innocence, and now provides lots of fond memories.

In those days, I had plenty of friends to play with. It was due in part to a willingness to go along to get along. I had a quiet confidence that other people noticed and were attracted to. Thanks to my mother, there were plenty of activities for me to stay busy with. Positive things like sports and stuff like that. I had not really fallen into that minefield of boy-girl relationships yet. Besides my old girlfriend Kay, with whom I had little contact since we had moved on to junior high school, and the girls on the block that we chased around with the regular amount of young horny tendencies, there were no girlfriends to speak of. So we used our youthful energy to play sports like organized and street baseball, basketball and football. Having the opportunity to learn how to be a team player, how to get along with my peers and to work together in a group for the greater good, were some of the lessons those men and that experience provided.

Therein lies the paradox of life in SSJQ. Everything seemed to be really cool on the exterior. When I look at how well we were provided for under those not so complimentary conditions, I am even more grateful for what we had as children. Our parents and the adults that were involved with our extra curricular activities provided relatively well for us, especially when you consider the obstacles. They did that while fighting off the psychological oppression that we all faced during those times. There were inconsistencies in the world, in my house and in my own head. Experience would come to be my major tool for learning about how to be a man, but there were opportunities abound for self-destruction. For instance, right on the corner or across the boulevard was all of the pain and suffering that I would ever want or need to experience. All I needed was to be curious enough to try it. All I needed to do was to be angry enough to not care. I had a choice and free will, even if both were limited by the reality of my environment. Like Javan said, "What a price we pay for experience, when we must sell our youth to buy it."

WHAT'S GOING ON?

...picket lines and picket signs,don't punish me with brutality, come on talk to me so you can see what's going on.
Marvin Gaye

Then came the summer of '69. I became a bit freer this particular summer. I was out of junior high and on to high school. I was kind of shy or at least reserved. I was certainly starting to feel the gap in my age with the girls I went to school with. I had more freedom to hang out and I was glad to be away from the drama at home. It was a fact that trouble could erupt at any time between my parents. By this time my father was progressing in his battle with alcohol and he and my mother were arguing with more regularity and venom. This summer I would grow up more than I could have possibly imagined, and in more ways than one.

It was the summer of Marvin Gaye and the question was "What's Going On?" The main answer to that musical question was drugs, joblessness and dead soldiers being shipped home to heartbroken families and a confused and discontented country. It was great music for a sad truth, and anyone that heard the way that Marvin laid out the state of the world in the powerful lyrics and moving music had to agree with that assessment.

This was certainly a time in our country's history when change was going to happen, one way or the other. We had already seen some great men murdered because their quest for human rights was incongruous with the political agenda of the powers that be. My father, who was the smartest man that I knew, had taken me to the March on Washington some years earlier. We were there when Dr. Martin Luther King gave his "I have a dream" speech on the great lawn. Things were beginning to shift and our generation was a part of making that shift happen.

At the '68 Olympics, there were two black fists raised in defiance of a world system that was still institutionally and legally discriminating against people who looked like me. Muhammad Ali was driven to take a stand against our country's involvement in Viet Nam by refusing to be drafted. Our government had to expect that there was civil unrest on the horizon, and that it had the potential to turn into an uprising. I am sure that they felt the people had to be controlled by any means necessary.

The baseball team that I had come to love and identify with, the New York Mets, was on its way to shocking the world with a run for the pennant and a world championship. I identified with them because they epitomized the underdog. That is what we were too. I was able to watch them grow from worst to first and to do it with them. Only we real fans had real hope of them winning, and even we did not see it happening as amazingly as it did.

Another taste of reality for me was when Cleon Jones, their star outfielder, was chastised on the field by his manager Gil Hodges. Then he was forced by then owner Joan Payson to apologize in the media for some off-the-field stuff that should have been a private affair between his family and the team. This was a terrible embarrassment for those of us who cared. It had not been that long since black ballplayers were allowed to play in Major League baseball, and it was a shame to see one of baseball's premiere players get that kind of treatment. It was like he was being flogged publicly. There was not only a lot of black and white in this world; there was also a whole lot of gray area that we had to work in. Cleon, understandably, had made the choice between leaving his high paid job and maintaining his public dignity, or kissing some major butt to keep his job and status. He chose the latter.

I understood how Cleon must have felt. In my neighborhood, I had the image of being an "all American" kind of guy, so I did what I could to protect that image. I was no angel though, and could have easily been put in a situation, like Cleon, where principles and desires meet head on. In that situation, which one would I choose? Like Muhammad Ali, would I stand up for what I believed, or would I acquiesce to keep or get what I desired? Time would give me plenty of chances to choose between the two.

I was not the only one trying to protect my image. I had turned 14 and was feeling grown, so I decided to get a summer job instead of going to camp as I had done the years prior. I guess there are no coincidences in how things seem to work out. I ran into some guys who would be a part of changing my life. They were guys that were trying to do the same thing as me. The fact is that we were young and should not have been doing some of the things we were doing.

The guys that I ended up working with that summer were running a youth organization that was centered on a basketball team. It was the best team in the neighborhood. Politicians and gangsters alike respected the youth organization that we ran with little or no resources. The least the city could do was to provide summer jobs for the ghetto youth. Because of that I was allowed to work with the Trotters of Jamaica for the summer as a Neighborhood Youth Corps employee. We did a lot of good in our hood. It was a learning experience for me in that it was my first job and it would serve as a bridge for me from junior high to high school. It is also when I started getting high on marijuana regularly, and had my first real meaningful experience with another girl.

I enjoyed getting high so that I could laugh a lot and so I could comfortably talk to girls. It is amazing how far that $40.80 we made working Neighborhood Youth Corps used to go! That is how much we used to make a week. That was more than I had ever earned. We were able to buy a pair of high-top black Converse sneakers, a pair of Jordache jeans, a pack of tube socks, a carton of cigarettes and still have plenty left to chip in on an ounce of pot for us to smoke until our next check. The six of us would get $40-$60 together to buy what we would need until our next paycheck. It never seemed to last long enough. So, in order for us to maintain, we learned where to buy (and sell) pot. We mostly bought, but we would sell a nickel and dime bags ($5/$10) or joints to our friends. I never mastered the selling thing, though. I could never seem to follow the Golden Rule—don't get high on your own supply. I guess this was our equivalent of business 101, a very special class given this way only in the school of hard knocks. I was happy to sign up for this elective.

It was important that we not let anyone know that we were getting as high as we were. After all, we were all barely teenagers. Our coach was a few years older than us and would have been in a great deal of trouble if anyone were to know. There were very few times that we played that we were not high. We were damn good and played extremely well as a team even if we were high. We hardly ever got beat and people loved to watch us play. I had never had as much fun playing basketball as I did playing with the Trotters of Jamaica.

We did not have to be in a gang because all of the gangs wanted to be like us. We spent everyday together, so I got to be extremely close with my teammates. For all intents and purposes, they had become my family. Being with them was a reprieve from the stress and embarrassment of the arguing that was going on at my house. Even if I was often the brunt of my teammate's jokes because of my having been skipped or using "big" words, I did not care. I still felt like I belonged because they trusted me enough to make me a part of the team.

DON'T PUSH ME

...don't push me cause I'm close to the edge—I'm
trying not to lose my head. It's like a jungle
sometimes it makes me wonder how I keep from
going under.
Grand Master Flash & The Furious Five

Getting high was fascinating. It made me happy and
was an escape from reality. That seemed like the
thing to do because reality could sometimes be
depressing to me. Besides, my own personal baby demons were
growing. The depths of my insights were growing right along
with those demons. The many discussions that I had heard
between my father and his best friend George had groomed
my mind to be able to read between the lines of the story
society was attempting to write for us. They had shot Dr.
King, John F. Kennedy and his brother Bobby, and Malcolm
X. They were vilifying Muhammad Ali for standing up for
his beliefs. The elusive "they" was messing it up for everybody.
I guess that suspending me for saying "damn" in math class
was small by comparison, but it changed my world. Thanks
to that old white haired math teacher Mrs. Kennedy and her
accomplice, the dean Mr. Muratore, for railroading me on that
one, I really took a butt whipping for that one indiscretion.
It was the first time my father had to beat me. It is not that I
did not merit punishment any earlier. I must have been quite a

frustration for my father. He would often try to communicate with me, but the more he tried the more I lied. I was afraid to stand up to him and tell him the truth. I was very much afraid of his reaction. I was sure that it would not be pleasant and based on what I had seen of my father's temper, it seemed better for everyone if I just lied about my actions or did not say anything at all. Watching me begin to set myself up to have the same kinds of dysfunctional attitudes and behaviors as my father had already acknowledged in himself had to be pretty frustrating for my father. I am sure that he must have felt as powerless over my actions as he was over alcohol.

I'll always love my mama. She brought me in this world (you only get one, you only get one, yeah). Moms did not take much from people either, especially concerning Pam or me. Both she and my father always wanted the best for me or Pam, and they would give me the benefit of the doubt in any questionable situation. I was a rebel in my heart and I really tested their resolve to be patient and loving parents, I know. I had told so many lies and even when I was caught red-handed doing something, I was not inclined to be truthful if it meant exposing myself to any consequences, whether those consequences were justified or not. As a way of trying to prepare me for the harsh realities of life in the way that she was conditioned to dealing with it, my mother told me that "It is their world, baby, and sometimes you may just have to go along to get along." I felt more inclined to try to change things. But I needed to find the courage to do something. Again though, it was wisdom my mother had and felt obligated to share with Pam and me. It was a truth that I understood and accepted as something that I would have to change about the world.

My sister Pam did not get into any of the kinds of stuff I was more than ready to explore. It was those differences in our behavior and appearance that made it easier for me to tease her about having been left on the steps of our house in a basket. It was not easy for her, either: she had the benefit of my growing reputation and the burden of it as well. With our peers it was to her benefit because I was known as a really good athlete and a really nice guy. The teachers in the schools I attended had a different take on my personality. They probably labeled me as a brat and a smart-ass with a lot of unrealized potential. Pam was wise enough that when she was given the choice to go to a different school and make her own way, she took it. It was a wise choice.

EASE ON DOWN THE ROAD

...don't you carry nuthin that might be a load, c'mon
ease on down, ease on down the road.
The Wiz

Working for the Trotters was my way to be a
part of something big and positive. We kept a
lot of young people out of trouble by running
basketball tournaments, giving bus trips and creating jobs for
youth. We kept our parks clean and stayed out of the streets.
We were community activists at the young age of 15. There
was a time when we were going to try to gain some political
clout by running one of my boys for a District Council seat.
We were smoking and selling pot all along the way. I did not
think that was the worst that could happen to a teenager in
SSJQ. Smoking pot was kind of normal to us. Most of the guys
I had grown up with thus far were into things like heroin and
methadone, so I was still pretty clean by comparison. Among
other things, these experiences taught me about survival.

It was around this time that I figured I would try to be
more forthright and honest about whom I was and what I
wanted. It took a great deal of courage for me to ask my father
for permission to smoke cigarettes at the age of 15. Everyone,
including me, was smoking already. We smoked on the way
to and from junior high school so getting permission would
just be a formality. It could mean the ability to smoke in the

house, maybe even in front of my parents. Being that my father smoked and we were not paying as much attention to the possibilities of cancer, I thought it possible Pops would grant me this wish. I hoped that it could be the opening for more honest dialogue in the future.

After all, I had not been caught with any of the harder drugs that my mother would warn us were out on the street. The chances for me successfully taking this step towards manhood were good enough for me to risk my father's wrath and ask for permission to smoke. I will never forget the response I got when I stepped to him while he was doing some yard work and very nervously inquired what his policy would be. He said that he would not give me permission to smoke because if he did I would soon be drinking, smoking reefer and then using heroin. I could not believe that he went there with me. It seemed unrealistic to think that just by smoking cigarettes I would end up mainlining dope! It did not happen that way for him and the millions of others that smoked cigarettes, did it? I could not understand how he knew it right then, but his response turned out to be quite prophetic. I can't even say it was a self-fulfilling prophecy, because I had been smoking pot regularly for some time already. I admit that cigarettes were the beginning of my addiction. They would be one of the last things I would have to pray that God would remove. Thank God that He relieved me of that habit.

When I first started hanging out with the Trotters, I was picked to move into the starting lineup because I had the God given gift of being able to jump really high, like out of the gym. Our coach, Dave, had a great eye for talent. He was unique in his ability to know just how to motivate each of his players. It seemed that his approach with me would be to challenge my desire and will.

I was more of a thinker, and though we had to play smart, there needed to be a kind of intelligence that would allow me to do things on the court as though it were second nature. You had to have game like that if you wanted to be respected on the courts of SSJQ. There were some real ballers around and they loved nothing more than to try to beat the Trotters. For that reason we practiced constantly. I had a whole lot to learn about playing "Trotter ball," though. The foundation to our game was built on dedication and teamwork.

I was still a little soft for the streets so I had to get tough. I did not have the killer instinct that would be needed to play with these guys and to be a winner. Winning was the tradition of the Jamaica Globetrotters and I would have to be groomed to step into it. Gaining and using the kind of bravado and confidence it took to win would be essential if I wanted to be able to hang out. This was not Inwood Street. I had branched out into the world. I would have to make a new name for myself. I was not sure what that name would be, but I was willing to toughen up. I had no real choice in my opinion. It is what we do when our backs are against the wall, right?

It was not only on the court that I would have to be toughened up. I was very sensitive and did not have the desire to fight back when being provoked or laughed at. I did not want to hurt anyone else's feelings, even if they were trying to hurt mine. I had enough of the arguing going on at the house. I was not sure that people could argue and still be friends. I needed to have some friends because I did not want to go home and I did not want to be alone. It was important that I got along with everyone.

Sometimes it seemed that there was a bit of jealousy or envy going on with our coach Dave and me. He had not graduated from high school and though he was a really smart and confident guy and he seemed not to even care about an education for himself. He pushed us to get good grades and would not let us play if we didn't. Yet here I was on track to graduate high school at 16 and feeling that Dave was a little harder on me because he was secretly envious. I was at the other end of the scholastic spectrum from Dave. As far as book smarts was concerned, I was the guy on the team that everyone looked to first. There were other guys like Ron and James Barfield were really intelligent and getting good grades, but I was in the highest grade. It was something that I could contribute to the crew. What I got from them was some street smarts and better use of my common sense. They made damn sure of that.

Many times we would hang out in the coach's room that he rented in the attic of a family over on 166th St. It was typical of the times—replete with a black light, lots of posters that glowed under the black light and a stereo that we would blast whenever possible.

This is usually where we would smoke and get really high. Sundays were the best times because we would start out at 7 am and run a few miles to the gym at the Naval Hospital in St. Albans. After a few hundred lay ups, 100 in a row from either side of the rim, we would run drills and full courts until our tongues were hanging. Those were the kind of practices that made us the best. When they were over, we would buy a few six packs of Budweiser, plenty of spiced ham and cheese and go to coach's place to chill. We would get real high and listen to all kinds of music like Earth, Wind and Fire, Chicago, The Isley Brothers, Isaac Hayes, Curtis Mayfield—oh man, the list goes on.

When we would leave coach's place, I would not want to go home. I really did not want to be there at my house for the next throw down. Besides, more times than not I was, as the Chilittes would sing "stoned outta my mind." I did not want to have to blow my high by going home. It was not that I was not cool and very good at hiding our altered state of mind from whomever I dealt with. I just wanted to enjoy the release, I guess.

Even though it was the sixties, and it was all about peace and love, I did not want to take the chance of finding out what most folks attitude towards teen drug use was going to be. Besides, I already knew how they felt about drugs. I had listened many times to my mother tell me about someone that we knew who was caught using or selling drugs. I would think to myself, if she only knew. So I knew it was no one's business what I was doing, especially if I wasn't hurting any one else.

Getting high was the real bonus of all we were doing. For me, it was the escape I was looking for. I could just float—float on—until it was time for us to wake up everybody, no more sleeping in bed, no more backwards thinking time for thinking ahead. The world won't get any better, than what it used to be. We got to change the world, just you and me.

BASKETBALL JONES

I got a basketball (love) Jones for you.
The Five Stairsteps

Of the six of us—the starting five and the coach—three of us lived closer to Sutphin Boulevard. George and Dexter lived on Dave's side of the tracks. The Barfield brothers, James, Ron and I walked home together many a day or night and I stopped at their house whenever I could. It got to be that I was there in their basement a great deal more than I was at home. Their family was warm and complete, and though I am sure they were not the Cosbys, it surely was peaceful.

James is the older of the two brothers and the one who was charged to take me under his wing. He was the other forward on the starting five and Ron was the center. I was the tallest of the three of us, and on the starting five. Height was not the final consideration as to what position we played. It came down to skills. James and I worked a little more closely so we became very close. I loved and admired Ron as well, but my relationship with "Bird" was different.

We called him "Bird" because of the way he could fly. I knew that I was jumping high too, but though James was a few inches shorter than I was, he was all over the rim. Bird had an assertiveness and competitiveness about him that reminds me of Michael Jordan. He was the guy I looked to pass to and listen to most. Watching the way we learned to play defense together was like watching a well-rehearsed, superbly choreographed play. It made you want to give a standing ovation. I learned a great deal from him about basketball and life.

His almost twin brother Ron was clearly the funniest and most innovative one in our crew. He had been on the honor roll for years and he kept us cracking up with the things he would say and do. James and I thought we would pee in our pants the night we were walking home, high as usual, from Dave's room at Miss Tina's house, and Ron started jogging in front of us. Suddenly, he jumped the short chain linked fence, and started spontaneously doing the bump with a big oak tree. Ron's dance with a tree that night was an instant classic prank that still ranks extremely high in the jokester's hall of fame.

Mrs. "B" and the rest of the family would provide the love and role models that I would draw from to live. There were four generations of women who lived in the Barfield family. Ms. Moore, or "Gran" as she is affectionately called, was the matriarch of this line in the family. I got plenty of opportunities to talk to Ms. Moore and she treated me just like one of the family. I would love to listen to her stories about Mr. Littman and his family. Mr. Littman was the white man whose family that Gran had worked for and taken care of for many years. Gran was happy about the way that they treated her as well. You could tell that by the way she beamed when she talked about the Littman family. She had been with the Littmans for a long time and had raised all of their children so they were like family to Gran. Any family of Gran's was bound to be all right with us.

They had a summerhouse at the beach that a proud Gran took us to visit one day. I think she was really happy to be taking us into the world that she spent so much of her time and energy living in. Gran certainly had a lot of energy. I was glad that she took me with her and treated me just like one of her own.

It was like I had angels all around me giving me just what I needed to keep pushing on. The day we went to the Littman's house I had really needed to get away from reality and the pressure of living in the city. The time we spent with Gran, digging for clams that we would later eat, was right on time. Gran looked on us with the loving gaze that only a grandmother can give as we laughed about the slimy texture of the clams. It wasn't like we had ever had them before. It was not the only thing new to me. I didn't have this kind of a relationship with my grandmother, so this kind of love was kind of new to me too.

Gran's daughter, Charlotte, is the mother of the family. I had affectionately taken to calling her "Mama." She is the one that makes things happen in that family. Mrs. "B" was a surrogate mother to a lot of the other kids and especially to me. She was a no nonsense kind of person that demanded respect. Though she was a short, small framed woman by the time I had met her, her spirit would begin to fill the room before she physically would enter it. I had heard stories of the cancer and TB that she had overcome years before. Those stories only added to the amount of respect that I had for the kind of courage that she displayed. It helped me understand the love, respect and admiration that her family had for her.

She would tell you how it T-I-S is, as she would say, and would do so with quickness. I respected her a great deal for the way she managed her family. It was an extended family with an open door for stragglers like me. If it true that it takes a village to raise children, then Mrs. Barfield must have believed it to be the way to live, because she certainly helped to raise me. Thank God for her love and protection. Without her hospitality I would have spent a lot more time in the less safe, more impressionable streets of SSJQ.

Mrs.B sure could cook. I ate more meals there than I care to admit. I would often be there at dinnertime and they were just too kind not to ask me if I wanted to eat. I was never ashamed enough to say no. So I became another mouth to feed. I would do whatever was necessary to not have to go home. Mrs. B's cooking was reason enough to hang out right there.

Her granddaughter Cynthia was a little older than James, Ron and I. She was more like Dave's age and she had two daughters of her own, making the four generations complete. "Simp" was my older sister, something else that I did not have at home. I had a few older female cousins that I had special relationships with, but Cynthia was my heart. She was sympathetic towards me. She would sometimes be the only one to try to rescue me when I would say or do something that would expose me as being sometimes timid and somewhat gullible. I was just learning how to play bid whist, and there was no mercy on me just because I was in the process. The best way to learn how to play bid whist is to get beat a few times.

Simp helped me to learn how to stand up for myself. I was the type who would not try too hard to defend myself when routinely being teased. Teasing can be cruel, but it is just what kids do to each other. Anyway, I was becoming a resourceful type of person. When I was being challenged by the ridicule of my peers, or backed into a corner, sooner or later I would come out swinging. I was developing character, but you could not have told me that then.

I probably knew as much about the Barfield family as I did my own. I watched their family evolve over time. When I first started hanging out at their house, Mr. & Mrs. Barfield, like all of the other adults in my life, were known to have a drink or two as grown folks do. It was quite amazing when they decided to stop drinking. Not long after, Mrs. B started attending church. I watched that transition with a strange curiosity. I knew the battles that my father was having with Mr. Booze. I did not know that anyone could or would stop drinking. I knew that drinking liquor could cause problems for those who got too drunk, too much, but I had never seen anyone stop for good. The only time we even had suggested it was possible was in jest. To see, up close and personal, someone who was actually defeating alcohol was amazing. As we began to drink more and more we would kid each other that there was a seat in AA just waiting for us. For me, that would turn out to be true.

I thought that the discipline that it took to stop drinking was miraculous. I was right. Everyone I knew was doing something to get high at least some of the time. Why "mama" would stop drinking, or the fact that she *could* stop drinking, planted a seed in my mind. I did not personally know anyone else who had successfully accomplished that feat. It was not something that I could see in my future, either. I just knew that I would die with a joint in my hand and a drink nearby. Somehow, knowing that it could be possible for a person to live without drinking was important for me to see.

My parents did not drink all of the time. There were plenty of times when my father would not be drinking. It seemed to be a chore for him to not drink. He was a different, much more sober, somber person without the drink. I think it hurt him not to have a little taste. I remember telling my friend Billy once when pops was on the wagon, that I was wishing he would jump off and take a drink so he could chill out and cheer up. He seemed to be white knuckling the situation. He would always comply with my secret wish and succumb to temptation. Then I would feel guilty for having prayed for it. The guilt was soon overwhelmed by the pain of watching helplessly as the man that I believe is the smartest, wisest and most loving person I have ever known, battle this vicious enemy. The seemingly uncontrollable urge to drink would be the albatross around my father's neck.

I'LL BE THERE

...build my world dreams around you, I'm so glad
that I found you. I'll be there with a love that's
strong, I'll be your strength—I'll keep holding on.
The Jackson 5

Soon, hanging out at the Barfield home would have
more benefits. The Trotters were going to recruit some
cheerleaders and one of the prospects lived on the same
block as Ron and James. There was a girl that lived on their
block and had grown up around his crew. Her name was
Nanette. I thought she was kind of cute and I was feeling like
we might be able to hit it off. She used to wear her hair in a big
Angela Davis afro that made her look like one of the Jackson
Five family. With her five brothers and two sisters, they had
the cast to try to be like them.

I had been kind of shy, but smoking pot was giving me
the kind of courage I needed to be able to say the things that
were on my mind. I was someone new for her to be around, so I
guess there was an attraction there for her too. We would have
plenty of time to get to know each other. Chemistry would
soon run its course.

When I smoked herb, I was able to say the things that
had been buried deep in the recesses of my heart. Most of
the time they were buried there behind a wall of shame and
insecurity. The walls of the fortress that held my emotions

were fortified by the bars of fear and guarded by all of the negative experiences that I had previously encountered when sharing my feelings and emotions with another. Those feelings and emotions were always there at the ready, waiting to escape. I guess that is why I used to cry so much.

The environment that we were living in was like a lake of fire. Only a ship built of courage would be able to navigate the lake. My ship would have to be built with some help. Getting to know Anne, and feeling like she might like me too, helped me to find some of that courage. Smoking pot made it easier to find. Together, I dreamed, we would build the ship and sail on a fantastic voyage. It would be like riding on the Enterprise, going where no man has ever gone before.

I wanted to know that I could have the kind of relationship like the ones I saw on TV. I knew that what was on TV was not necessarily real, but the concept of a happy relationship or really just being in love had to be a real possibility. Otherwise, why go on living? There had to be more to this life than what I was seeing in reality. On TV and in the movies, there was always a happy ending. Where were the Cosby's or the Brady's, Cleaver's or Rob and Laura Petrie now?

***

I spent a lot of time hanging out with the Trotters and over the Barfields', and I got to see Anne often in both places. She was the one I was destined and privileged to fall in love with. Nanette was crazy in love with me and she showed it in every way. My nose was wide open too. It was that intense puppy love that felt so grown. Thinking about her had me singing songs like the Chilites—"Stoned outta my mind" and Heatwave's "Always and Forever." At the tender age of 14 I felt that I had found a love that my heart had been longing for. I would not have to shop around anymore. This was it.

I was staying away from home and in the streets as much as possible. I lived with my mother and father for sure, but I was going to raise myself as best I could without much more input from them. I was glad to love them and to accept any help they could provide, but I would not expect them to be there for me at all. It was time for me to grow up and make my way in the world. Even though I was still a little short on street smarts, I was learning how to get by, and I had plenty of angels to help.

Anne and her family were a new addition to my life. They became a part of my village, you know, the one it takes to raise a child. The strategy for rearing us, though unspoken, was very evident and relatively effective. The parents would keep us at arm's length and somewhere in sight. They pretty much knew where we were at all times. Most of the time we were there at the house.

With as much time as I spent with Anne at Ron and James' house, we had plenty of time to get to know each other. She really knew how to take care of me. Anne was the one that I shared my quiet desperation with. Many an evening she would go to her home just across the street from the Barfields' place, and bring me food and comfort. The food was from the table of her mother and father and 7 siblings. The comfort would come in many ways. It was comforting to know that she cared that much and was willing to show me.

Her father, Rodman, had been an accomplished musician who had played with many of the jazz greats of his time. Now, he was basically working and taking care of his family. They were not rich by any means, but there was always a loving invitation to join them for dinner. It was not pity or anything. They all just knew that I was spending a lot of time in their homes and around their kids. They seemed to really like me too. The feeling was mutual. Many times Anne would wrap a plate that her mother had made and sent to me while I was down the block at Ron and James.

Mrs. Whitman, Anne's mother was a saint. Not the unapproachable kind of saint that seems too good to really be true. She was real enough. What she had to do to raise her 8 children in the war zones of The Bronx and now their home in SSJQ is what qualifies her for sainthood. How she was able to do that and still be as active as she was in the community was inspiring. She and Mr. Whitman had been married for a long time and their older children had long since left the nest. Even with the effect the love and dignity their relationship had on all of their children, alcohol had taken its toll on their family as well.

In the Whitman household, while the insanity did not reach the frantic level that it sometime reached at my house, the effect was still evident. Well, it did get crazy there too, sometimes. One thing that seemed to be common with the men of that generation was that they all were dealing somehow with the sometimes reluctant resignation to the lives that they were living. It is not that they were unhappy. It just seemed that they all had greater potential and that they were being stunted by the social oppression of the day.

Most of them had, to some extent, achieved the American dream. They had houses and cars and were taking care of their families. They had good jobs with benefits and came home every night. It didn't outwardly matter that they had had great dreams and hopes for themselves and their children. There was no reason that they should not be able to have a few drinks at night or on the weekend if they wanted. If they got a little drunk, so what? They were doing what they had to, so they should be able to do what they wanted, too.

Everyone was doing it and their parents had probably done the same thing. The problem is that underneath the drinking was a way to forget about the responsibility of raising a black family in America. Liquor was an anesthetic used on this battlefield of life. It was used to dull the sting of having to do all of what they did while dealing in a system that was somewhat hostile towards them. The whole thing seemed to be testing their resolve. It was a way for their generation to reconcile with the youthful ambitions and dreams that were now slowly fading to black. That reality seemed to create an underlying attitude of silent despondency. Which one came first, despondency or the drink? I don't remember, but as a team they made a formidable adversary.

MOVE ON UP

...so hush now child and don't you cry, your folks might understand you by and by. Remember your dreams are your only schemes-so keep on pushing, take nothing less-not even second best and do not obey. You must have your say; you can pass the test...Move on up!

I know that my mother would be there for me whenever she could, but she was so busy working to provide a roof over our heads and some independence for herself, that she really did not have the time to try to keep up with me. She was a beautician, and that meant long, erratic hours on her feet and being available for her clients mostly every day. Ma had worked at other jobs after coming north at the tender age of 16. Mom often talked about how relatively well off she was down in Charleston; it is a wonder why she felt the need to leave home at such a young age. She moved to a completely different lifestyle, one that was much more challenging than the one she had left.

While living in Charleston with her mother and stepfather, my mother had it pretty good. Her stepfather was an entrepreneur who had a store and other real estate. He was able to provide very well for his family and my mother enjoyed the fruits of his labor. She would eat whatever she wanted from two stores in the neighborhood without a care because her parents had accounts there. Moving to New York had proved to be a real test of her character, a test that she passed with flying colors. After a career at the telephone company was shortened by my birth, my mother was able to reinvent herself as a beautician. She figured that the change would give her more time to raise a family, and still allow her the opportunity to maintain some level of independence. Both of those things were very important to her.

Working as a beautician and trying to keep up with Pam and me was a challenge for her, too. Often she would have to work late and long, taking breaks only to check on us and make sure we were alright. Pam sometimes called Moms on the job to tell on me because I was trying to either boss her around or tease her. My mother had to become adept at running things at the house while being at the shop.

Between working any one of the swing shifts and drinking, my father did not have time to keep up with me. He had never really seemed to have the kind of time to take more of an interest in my athletic ability. I guess I could have been upset if I thought a father should have more time for his son. At the time I was just glad that he was not trying to keep up with me so I could have the freedom I wanted. My father was the smartest and wisest man I have ever known. There would have been very little, if anything, that I would have been able to pull on him. Pops was uncanny in the way he would know what I was going to do, most times even before I did!

Pops obviously was no athlete himself, at least not so I would ever know. We did not even talk about sports that much, and when we did you could tell that it was a somewhat clumsy attempt by him to develop a relationship with me by coming into my world. He seemed somewhat ill equipped to create that kind of a relationship. It was as if he had never had that kind of relationship before so he only knew how to love me with the tools that he had. That would be just fine with me.

My father had grown up working on the farm, something I came to know he resented. So I guess sports weren't a part of his repertoire and it was the major part of mine. All I wanted to do was to play, and he knew it. I wondered if he ever he had the chance to be a kid and play the way I did. He supported me and rooted for me all the time, even if he did not get to come to many games. He was always asking how I was doing and he had a willing ear. Dad would listen to my accounts of the games and I was happy to share it with him. It was the way that we forged a bond between us.

My dad had to work a lot of different shifts as a New York City Housing cop. Sometimes he would "moonlight" as a cab driver so that he could make the extra money we needed to maintain the middle class life that he and my mother had carved out of the American dream. The few times that he did come to a game that I was playing in I remember distinctly.

One memory that stays with me is when I was playing in the little league all-star game. There were six teams in each division and we would play against each other during a 10 or 12 game regular season. Then the coaches would choose the best players from all of the different teams to play against other leagues and their best. Our quest was to get to the Little League World Series held annually in Williamsport, Virginia. We never made it to the World Series, but we beat plenty of teams trying to get there. We played many exciting games and made many an unexpected late inning comeback. There was one game that I was glad he was there to see me play in. I remember three things about that game. I remember him reading a copy of the Amsterdam News in between innings while we where playing the game, as if he were either uncomfortable about how he should act at a baseball game and not sure about how much attention to give the game and me. I also remember that he was not drunk for which I was relieved.

The fact that I hit a home run in that all-star game that he attended was unbelievable. It was right out of the script for a movie. That ball must have been aided out of the park by the baseball gods. When I hit it, it screamed off of my bat like it was going to be a double in the gap between the center and right fielders, but stayed in the air long enough to clear the makeshift outfield fence made of rope. Hey, this was the SSJQ. We did not have the kinds of well manicured, fenced baseball fields that they had in the white neighborhoods, but we kept them up just fine. I remember that when I was rounding the bases after hitting the home run, my father was standing and cheering and yelling, "That's my boy, that's my boy!!" The way he was beaming with pride made me feel complete. It was one of the few times I would see him drop his veil and show some kind of emotion towards me other than disgust or confusion. It is not that I did not feel loved by him. I really made it hard for him to get closer to me. It seemed that he and most men of his generation had a different way of showing their love.

Everything that I was doing in my life when I was acting out was an attempt to get the attention and affection from my father. It is not that he did not want to give me love and affection. That was certainly not the case. Since the time that Roy and Lou realized that the girl they thought they were going to have was really me, my father was as proud and hopeful of me as a father could be. I think that in some ways my father wanted to have a happy family life, but he did not seem to have the experience from which to draw. He had the love, but did not have the tools, and it was just one of the many contradictory emotions that created the cacophony inside his soul that was quieted only by drinking. So whenever Pops was trying to talk to me and understand why I behaved the way I did, confusion and disgust were the things that I saw in his face. That is the emotion that I saw most often directed towards me when I was going through my rebellious behavior in elementary and junior high school. It was the emotion I felt as I was trying to understand why I was so angry and why I did the things I would do. He would ask why and I would lie. It was a story that he would not buy. Despair was the emotion he felt for himself and I believe he may have been perplexed by his inability to tell me that he loved me. Or did he?

So, by the time I had met Anne and my other girlfriend, marijuana, I was glad to be able to have the kind of time to devote to developing a relationship with the both of them. It would be imperative that I have the kind of time that to share with them in order to get my point across. The point was that I needed to be loved and I wanted to be able to laugh. I needed to be able to tell someone that I loved him or her without being perceived as soft. It was important for me to have the kind of relationship that I did not have at home, nor did I even see at home. Unconsciously, I looked for a love that I could call my own. That was my plan.

Besides, the fun experiences of being a teenager with new found freedom was enough to keep my young ass in the streets as long as possible. Thinking that I would come home and have to deal with all of the fussing and fighting that could potentially be going on just gave me more reason to stay gone. I was playing ball, getting high, chasing girls and making money. If not for the drama between my daddy and my mama my life would have been as perfect as a young black man growing up in the SSJQ could be. Even with those challenges, things were good.

***

Some of my greatest pain came from having to call the cops on my own parents. There was always a lot of embarrassment and emotional torment the shame I felt when I would come home to the police, flashing their lights in front of my house. My mother and father would argue so violently sometimes, that my sister and I had no choice but to call the cops. I remember the time when he and my mother did battle and in her effort to keep him from leaving the house she pulled a knife on him and dared him to leave. It was as if she was saying that she did not believe that he was going out drinking with the boys, and even if he was, he needed to be spending some time at home with the family. She had been on the wrong side of one of those arguments prior to this episode, so the knife was more for self-defense. She knew that though Pops had little or no intent on hurting her, there was no real telling what would happen in a scuffle. I guess Ma was willing to put it all on the line believing that it was the liquor that was making pops so irrational towards her.

My mother and I did not see eye to eye on most things during those days and that was mostly because I had a need to be free and she needed me to love her. My mother was very protective, and I did not want to be protected. My mother and father would argue like they had done many times before. I would be torn between wanting to adhere to the verse in the Bible that admonished a good God fearing young man to honor thy mother and thy father, and cussing them both out for being so irrational and vicious towards each other. Of course, I had read the script for the movie that we were living, and the script called for the son to protect his mother first and foremost. I had no problem with playing my role, but my father was stronger, smarter and had a gun. Besides, most of the time I identified with his desire for freedom and silently rooted for Pops to prevail if for no other reason that if he was gone there would be some peace.

So when Mom pulled the knife on my father and made it clear in no uncertain terms that she'd really rather he stayed home that night, I knew there was going to be a problem. Pops was not the kind of guy that liked to be pushed around or told what to do. Going out and having a few drinks was something he had to do. He was the funniest guy that I knew when he was drinking and had a great wit. Dad was very intelligent, but there only seemed to be a very limited number of ways this scenario would end.

I remember Mom sitting there in front of the door with the steak knife in her hand. The two of them seemed to be negotiating the outcome with no compromise evident. The next thing I know, Pops was holding the gun on moms and she is holding the knife on him. The time had come for life to see what I was made of. It was up to me to head off this Mexican standoff.

It is all a blur now. Part of that is my mind shutting down the same way it did when the situation was unfolding. The mind will do that to protect us from overloading, I've heard. I do remember stepping in front of the gun that he had pointed at my mother in an attempt to diffuse the altercation. I remember that tactic working and feeling extremely bitter that I had been put in that situation. The last thing I would have thought I would have to do is to look down the barrel of my father's .38 caliber service revolver. I am sure it surprised them both that I would do such a thing. They were surprised enough to come to their senses long enough to put down their weapons. I had to yell and cry and generally lose my mind to do it. Afterwards, I lay in my bed and cried myself to sleep, on my knees and rocking my head in the pillow. I would rock myself to sleep like that often to shake off the fear and tension while trying to go to another world. Pops did not go out that night, but there was no episode of "Leave it to Beaver" being lived in our house that night or at any other time.

As drunk as father (and mother) would get, it is still a testament to the Creator and Her Grace that I am here to tell the story.

THANK YOU

I want to thank you for letting me be myself again.
Sly & The Family Stone

That is why I really did not want to be at home. I did not want to leave my sister Pamela there to deal with whatever may have happened, but she would have to fend for herself. It was not that she was in any kind of direct danger physically from what my parents were doing. I had no real gauge of how it was affecting her emotionally. I know that it just kind of worked out that I needed to be doing my own thing.

I had a couple of places that I could hang that would allow me to have fun, maintain my image, get high all the time and if I played my cards right I could finally get some real sex. It had been since fourth grade since I had really "made love" to anyone. How strange is it that a teenager would be so concerned with sex and drugs? I guess that once you get some, you are never the same again. It was just another day in the hood.

I had tried to have sex with a girl when we were in junior high school. There were times when we would play hooky from school and go to hooky parties or to the Lost Battalion, a gym on Queens Boulevard. We would go to that gym because we could play basketball there, all day, and never be questioned as to why you were not in school. It was a safe haven for hooky players.

If you were lucky, you could get your girlfriend, or anyone's girlfriend to go to one of these hooky parties. I guess the sexual revolution that America was experiencing during the '60s and the '70s helped cause our premature thirst for sex; that, and those wild hormones. Somebody would have the heart to invite other students to their house, figuring that their parents would be at work all day. I could never take that kind of chance with my parents or my house. I was afraid to get caught in mine or anyone else's house, with a girl no less. If you were going to get caught doing something you were not supposed to be doing, that may have been the thing worth trying. So eventually I did go for it when the opportunity arose.

One time, I went to a hooky party with my god brother and his girlfriend. His girlfriend had a friend that liked me and was going to hang out, so I was invited. It was a given that they were going to be doing their thing sexually and obviously it wasn't their first time. This would be my first real opportunity to share a sexual experience since being in junior high school.

It was a good news/bad news story, to be sure. We all waited until our parents had gone to work and then we sneaked back to the house where we would stay until it was time for us to be out of school. We all sat around together for a little while before Wayne and Janet went into Wayne's room and closed the door. I was kind of shy, but much more horny than I was shy, so I was really happy that my "date" was willing to lie down with me.

That always seemed like the greatest honor was the fact that a young lady would pull her panties down and give me the opportunity to not only be close but to be inside her. This was an overwhelming gesture of trust and I learned that kissing and telling was a violation of that trust. I had learned how to keep things to myself from the relationship that I had with my parents. I would not tell my mother anything for fear she would use it to get what she wanted. I would tell my father a lie or nothing at all for fear of what he would say or think. So, keeping things to myself was nothing new to me. I could be discreet.

The good news was that is that finally someone liked me enough to trust me with their all and all. The bad news is that I was inexperienced and she was a virgin. That is a combination for frustration. I think I got close to penetration. I know that it was a lot like the sexual relations that I had with Kay back in fourth grade. Was this the real deal with sex? Don't get me wrong. I enjoyed the experience a great deal except for the embarrassment of not knowing where to put it in. I was grateful for the chance to try. Not that the sexual experience was so satisfying. It was more that I felt like I was worthy of love. That is what was being shared more than anything else, a feeling of being wanted. That was very satisfying to my young and fragile ego.

That satisfaction did not last for long. My ego and image were going to be destroyed if I could not perform. I had no problem getting an erection. When you are twelve or thirteen, the last thing you have a problem with is an erection. It is more of a problem hiding an unexpected woody, and having to hide an obvious bulge in one's pants was a pretty common occurrence. Sometime when the wind blew, I would get hard from the excitement.

I did not even know what the problem I was having in penetrating my young virgin lover was until I confronted my more experienced godbrother Wayne with the situation. I had to ask him. I did not want the opportunity to come and go without doing my best to make her feel as good as I could about what we were doing. After all, it was not like it was a secret from Wayne or Jackie. We all knew why we were there and he was a year and a half older and much more experienced than I. I thought he may have the answer.

After he explained it to me I did not feel as inept. It was her first time. She had blessed me with the honor of being the first real sexual partner she would have. I wish that I had known what I was doing. I was never satisfied with my performance that day and felt kind of embarrassed about my lack of experience.

I continued to pursue a relationship with the young lady and we were boyfriend and girlfriend for most of the school year. It was evident that I had a great deal to learn about male-female relations. I did like the feeling of being loved and wanted to be able to trust someone enough to give my love without fear of being hurt. I had never had what I know now as unconditional love. To me, even my relationship with my mother was not one of unconditional love. I had my doubts that it would be possible. These were tough times for the two of us. I was trying to learn how to be her son and learning how to be a person. In the process I realized that my parents did not have any experience with being parents either.

Even at that young and tender age, I had already begun to build a fence around my emotions. I had been such a crybaby as a kid and was teased a lot for being one too. It wasn't a cool thing to do and it could have been much more troublesome for me if it had not been for the way that people seemed to like me.

As a natural function of being a kid in the hood, or anywhere else, you have to put up with a certain amount of teasing from your peers. There were kids around my way and that went to school with me that were really good at finding your weaknesses and exploiting them publicly. Given the opportunity, some guys would dog you out. There were some kids that would talk about you on the bus to school so bad, that they would have everyone on the bus laughing at you. I knew that if it were me that was the brunt of this kind of abuse, it would hurt my feelings bad enough to make me cry. Crying wouldn't get you any more sympathy, either. Actually, it would be the thing to give a guy who was at first just a comedian enough courage to want to fight you or chase you home. When that happened on the block, my mother would try to make me go back out there and stand up for myself, but I never wanted to fight or even hurt anyone else's feelings. I would not try to verbally battle with those that were moving themselves up in the pecking order by walking over me.

So, by the time I started hanging out with Anne, I was ready for another shot at love, or my interpretation of it. If she decided to be with me that way, I was going to get it right this time. The world seemed like a cold place and as I got older, I became more guarded with my feelings. By the time I had begun to hang out and work with the Trotters, I had learned how to hide the buttons that controlled my emotions. I was learning how to not take myself so seriously. I had learned how to not let people know what or how I was feeling. The ironic thing is that not knowing what I felt was more intriguing and frustrating to those same people, including my parents, who had gotten quite comfortable with pushing my buttons. There was always a great deal of expectations for what I would become because of my intelligence and ability. The main flaw in my young and still forming personality was that I lacked self control. The universe was teaching me a lesson. I would have to toughen up if I was going to survive in my family, in my neighborhood, and in the world. I did, and by the time this particular summer rolled around, I was almost finished erecting the brick wall that was to enclose my fragile emotions so effectively that the only time they would see the light of day would be under most extreme circumstances. The pressure would have to build up so much that when my emotion did rear its head, it would show up as either one of two things— anger or love.

I was glad to have new friends on the team we called the Trotters, but they were products of the same environment as the others who had tormented me before. They did their teasing under the guise of trying to toughen me up, and supposedly with love, but to me it felt the same as always. It caused me to be really happy about the two things that began to fill the deep and expanding void that filled my heart with loneliness. That summer I opened my heart to the two loves that would rid me of any need for insecurity and loneliness. With these two loves, I would not have to ever be alone and angry. I could be loved, admired and very happy under almost any circumstance. It was that summer that I fell head over heels for my two new and all encompassing loves, marijuana and Anne.

SEXUAL HEALING

...ooohh, I'm hot just like an oven—I need some
lovin'...when I get that feeling, I need sexual
healing.
Marvin Gaye

So, by the time I was getting close enough to Anne to
start thinking I might be getting some sex, I was truly
ready for love. We seemed to hit it off and except for the
fact that she was the third daughter and seventh child of nine,
there was nothing to fear. I thought her oldest brother might be
someone I would have to reckon with if I did his sister wrong,
but I had no intention on doing that at the time. It got to where
we were seeing each other every day and doing the things that
young lovers do. The Barfield brothers had girlfriends that
were cheerleaders too, and we all were smoking pot together
and having big fun. It was the best of times, it was the worst
of times. Just another paradox of living our teenage lives in the
'60s & '70s in the contradiction of the United States, and more
specifically—in the South Side of Jamaica Queens.

We spent a great deal of time in Ron & James' basement
after we got closer to the girls. When we began to play ball
together, we spent a great deal more time playing ball than
anything else. As time went on and we became more involved
with the softness and passion that was available with the girls,
the proportion of time spent playing ball with the sweaty,

testosterone charged guys as opposed to chasing the sweet taste and aroma of the girls slowly shifted. We were just as likely to be listening to Marvin Gaye with the girls, as we would be across the tracks coolin' out with the fellas and listening to The Funkadelics.

The Barfields had the blessing of having an extended family that vibrated through the maternal lineage that included four generations. There was warmth that ran through their family that made it really easy to get consumed in their hospitality. I had taken to calling Mrs. Barfield "Mama" and felt like I could really trust her to be honest with me if I needed to share with someone. She certainly kept us out of more troubling experiences by allowing us all to hang out in the basement with her sons. At least if we were there where she could see us, or at least hear us, the chance of us getting beat up, shot up or cut up were diminished. All of those things were very much a possibility in SSJQ.

So, with all of the time that I was spending at Ron & James' house I got to see Anne mostly everyday. The more that I saw of her the more comfortable I felt to share myself and let my guard down around her. I began to trust her and was able to show my vulnerability to a certain degree. I did not take the brick wall guarding my emotions and feelings down, but I cut a hole in it to see if the fire was still burning. There was a fire burning alright, but it was not the fire fueled by my fears of the pain created by the cruel and unsympathetic world. This fire was created by the passion that burned in my heart. I longed for a love that would envelop me in its safe and protective bubble so that I could float around in this hell I saw the world as being, without having to feel the pain and suffering I had previously experienced.

Some would call it puppy love, but it felt like the big

dogs were barking in my heart. That was not the only part of my anatomy that felt like it was howling either. Anne and I were spending a lot of time together and were considered to be boyfriend and girlfriend by our friends and teammates, parents and anyone else that knew us. We knew that we had something special going and we were both feeling like we were ready for the next step. Well, I know I was ready to chase some kitty. It looked like I was about to catch some too. Either that or the pussycat was going to catch me. Why must I be like that, why must I chase the cat, nothing but the dog in me.

SUMMER MADNESS
Kool & The Gang

Near the end of the summer my parents decided they were going to go on a weekend trip to some Army fort on the beach in New Jersey. My parents were always taking me places. Some of the time I would not want to go. That is usually when I had the most fun. I had been spending a great deal of time away from home. My folks must have thought it would be a good chance to meet my new friends Ron and James, my new "girlfriend" Anne and for us all to get away from the battleground of the SSJQ for a couple of days. The fellas and I thought it would be an opportunity to be alone with our girlfriends. I was sure that this would be my chance to finally get me some of that yum yum I had been dreaming about all summer.

Anne had me right where she wanted me I guess. It was plain to me that one day we would consummate the relationship. It is just that if the day was not that very day, then it was at least one day too late. My testicles must have begun to change shades to a wild shade of blue by the time we took that trip together. She was making me wait for the opportunity. So I waited. After all, I did not know how I would perform when given the chance. I had not had a whole lot more experience since the virgin episode. I was going to need some courage to make it happen right. I really wanted to have a pleasurable experience and that meant bringing pleasure to her. It was not as much an ego thing as it was a statement about the kind of person I wanted to be. There was something really important to me about being kind, loving and considerate, especially inside a relationship.

We had chipped in on an ounce of reefer to take with us. There must have been about ten of us kids, five guys and five girls, including my sister and a few of the neighbors from the block. The parents were doing their thing, drinking and socializing while we enjoyed the freedom of the wide-open spaces, grass and trees. I would like to say the air was fresh, but this was New Jersey and even then there was always some pollution there. It seemed fresh because it was scented with the smell of salt water spraying that semi-deserted army barracks by the beach. It was a relatively clear day and visibility was good. Good enough for us to see the group of parents and for them to see us even though we were separated by over 150 yards of open field.

We were having fun and looking forward to more. We were going to spend the night in some old army barracks and the parents were all going to be across the old training field in a trailer over 300 yards away. This was finally going to be my opportunity to share some private and intimate moments with the girl that I now loved. Well, I loved her as much as a wounded puppy could love or trust anyone. I certainly loved her enough to want to spend an evening of passion together as a culmination of so many stolen moments of limited passion. My passion was only limited by how far Anne would allow me to go. This day, I thought, would be a special day unless something really drastic happened.

Something drastic almost did. Up until then, we had all maintained an air of innocence around adults, though I am sure that they must have suspected otherwise. It was imperative that they did not find out that we were drinking, drugging and trying to have sexual relations. My father was a cop, and even though he drank and was a lot of laughs to be around when he did drink, we did not want him to be on our case about anything, especially our smoking grass. Somehow that is exactly what almost happened that day.

We were walking away from all of the parents on our way to have our own adventures. I am sure they were just as happy to get rid of us so that they could laugh, curse and enjoy a few drinks, as we were to go on our merry way. They cussed around us kids anyway, except my mother who rarely did curse. I sensed that the adults wanted privacy as much as we did. The fact that they were going to let all us kids stay together over night was an indication of either their insanity or their plan. The girls were supposed to stay somewhere other than with us, but the moon was full and my father snored extremely loud. He actually snored loud enough for us to hear him across the field many yards away. It would not be hard for them to get rid of us, not at all. It would not be hard for us guys to sneak our way in the moonlit field to the place where the girls were supposed to be sleeping.

***

We had an ounce of some good weed and a lot of space and time to enjoy it. It was just what I would need to get us both in the mood for a night of sexual exploration. This would finally be the day we would go all the way. We had some music playing on a tape recorder. It was the Ojays singing "Bad Luck"—that's what you got, that's what you got. Just then someone asked where the herb was. At that moment I realized that I had left it in my royal blue Trotter jacket that just happened to be back over where the parents were. Just when I turned around to jog back over and get it, I saw my father with my jacket in his hands. He seemed to be raising it up high and looking in the pockets. All of us kids were looking at him by then and we all held our collective breaths waiting for the other shoe to drop. It was a moment frozen in time. It was as if the whole seen was happening in slow motion.

I could barely move from that spot. I did not know which way to run. I had to decide whether to run as fast as I could toward the jacket and my father in order to try to retrieve the jacket and the herbs before they were confiscated. If that were to happen all of us would be put on house arrest and there would be no way to have any fun after that. Or should I start and keep running the other way to a new life where I would never have to face the investigation. Investigation and interrogation was sure to follow any discovery of drugs, and after all was said and done, that is what marijuana is. If my father found our an ounce of primo weed that we had planned to consume that day it would be a devastating turn of events, especially in light of my possibilities for love.

The thought of not getting the sex that I had waited for so long to share was incomprehensible and the idea of not being able to consummate our new love paralyzed me with fear. We were 15 or so and could not afford or get a hotel room, and her family was so large that someone was always at home. Here was my best chance for love and I was going to lose it if we were to be busted. I would lose major cool points all the way around. It was not that often that my friends would come into my world and I did not want this episode to end so tragically.

I thought about that feeling of togetherness that I had been looking for all of my life and it seemed that I was so close to actually having that for myself with Anne. The thought of not getting the chance to experience that overwhelmed the fear that I felt about getting busted with the herb. I started running back towards my jacket and my father as fast as I could. I could not tell whether or not pops had discovered the pot or not, but lack of sex had surely made me brave. I was going to get that herb and that sex that night no matter what. So with my heart in my mouth, I made that 150 yard run hoping that the gods would smile on me just this once. If the gods would spare me the embarrassment, disappointment and lost opportunity this one time, I would gladly pay them back on another day.

The gods must have heard my prayer and took pity on my young blue balls. To this day I don't know if my father did not see the fat bag of weed in my pocket that day, or if he decided that he did not want to bust up either party with the drama that would have ensued. As a housing cop he surely must have dealt with situations like this before. The type of guy he was left room for the possibility that he chose the lesser of two or three evils. Maybe he just did not feel or see the bag and the pipe in the pocket. I know that it surely looked to us like he put his hand right in the pocket and was holding it up so as to let us know that he knew it was there.

He chose not to say anything to us and I felt that it was a good course of action, or non-action. The relief I felt was indescribable. It was still looking good for me to get next to Nanette and we were all going to get high and have some fun in the sun. That was among the best quality pot I ever had. I think it was enhanced by the drama. It turned out to be one of the most exciting nights of my young life. Having narrowly escaped certain disappointment through God's Grace, I turned my attention back to my new girlfriend. The parents had planned for the guys and girls to sleep in separate barracks. This was supposed to go down while the parents were sleeping in a trailer some 200 yards away. The full moon and my father snoring would be all we needed to have enough cover for the maneuver that night.

I remembered the last time I had the opportunity and the pleasure of having sex. This time was going to be different all right. I am pretty sure that it was her first time having sex. That is what she told me and I believed her. This time I was able to find the right place to put it. I could not control myself when I got there. In mere minutes, or less, I had reached the climax that had taken years to achieve in my mind. The feeling was one of extreme ecstasy. It was different from what I had experienced any other time. I had grown up in more ways than I knew. I wanted to make sure my partner was pleased too, even though my inexperience showed that I had much more to learn. At least I had the important part. The thing that has always come natural is a desire to please. It would be true of all my relationships, but I would go to almost any lengths to sexually please the women in my life.

I am not quite sure what one would call whatever I had been doing before when I thought I was having sex. This was really my first time having grown up sex. I experienced an orgasm this time. It came so quickly that it felt like there was something else I needed to do to please my mate. I felt like I had cheated her. It was going to take some time for me to get used to this kind of passion and yet maintain some kind of control. That was an oxymoron and I guess it was going to take some practice to be able to do. Anne and I made a pact that night to stay together forever. After all, how long could forever be? Forever ever, forever ever?

***

We spent plenty of time getting the sex thing down to a science. We both got to be very good at it after awhile. We went out of our way to get daily practice. The relationship needed work, though. Somehow, it was beginning to take on some of the same qualities as the relationship my parents had. I had sworn to never let that happen to me. It is amazing how that happens. You swear to yourself and others that you will never make the same mistakes as your parents and then you become them. Even if you do not actually repeat the same behaviors, most people certainly have to be conscious of not doing so.

Anne and I shared many years of love and experiences while growing up. It seemed that we would be together forever, just like we had vowed to each other before we decided to overlook what we had been taught was God's plan to have sex after marriage. I thought it very possible that we would be together forever, so logic and our hormones seemed to justify our sexual behavior. We were very young, though. Our attitudes about relationships were being formed subconsciously by our feelings, and more importantly, by the things that we saw happening in our world. The influences ranged from the free love mindset of society, to the "do as I say, not as I do" attitudes of our parents. Social pressures had developed situations that lent itself to extended families, both known and unknown, role reversals where women, especially Black women, were taking on the roles, responsibility and demeanor of the father. This angered many Black men who found it demeaning and discouraging that Black women would take the opportunities we had all fought for, and use it to act superior. It was also evident that Black men would have more obstacles to overcome in order to achieve the same level of social success. In a very real way, the friction that the changing society caused in the Black family was, and still is, a contributing factor to the way we behave sexually and the way we create relationships. It has always been difficult, at best, for Black folks, in particular, to reconcile our reality while attempting to assimilate European cultural behavior. We have had to deal with the effects of racism while denying that it has any actual affect on how look at sexual relationships and the consequences in our families. In that regard, Anne was not wrong for developing the Eurocentric female attitude of wanting "Prince Charming" to ride in on a white horse and be her "officer and a gentleman." She expected monogamy and felt justified in feeling possessive of her mate, which happened to be me. After all, that is what we had been taught was the right thing to want. Every aspect of American society perpetuates that view, even if it is not the way that most of the American society actually lives. I, on the other hand, believed that each person's body is his or her own, to share with whom ever they please. Sure, there are values and morals that we need take into account before we actually do jump into bed with another human being, but those decisions should be made out of love and integrity, not fear. If the truth be told, there are a great deal of secrets about sexual behavior and paternity in our community. Though men and women often see things very differently, there is one thing that I believe we have in common. Everyone really just wants to be loved. Is that so wrong?

Anyway, it seemed that Anne and I had reached that point of our relationship where we would have to come to some kind of reconciliation of our opposing viewpoints and how that would take into consideration our ability to deal with our emotions. I was intent on being free to do whatever my heart desired, yet I was willing to be respectful of our relationship and Nanette's feelings. My hope was that I would be able to be honest about it all without disrespecting the privacy of another. Her attitude about the relationship was not unlike that of most of her peers and predecessors. She expected total "fidelity," or at the very least to be lied to in the event of human frailty. It was really very confusing to be a "free thinker" that was trying to be respectful of her position. I loved Anne, but I was forming my own principles about life, and my experiences with watching the relationships of my parents and others had made an impact on me. My innate desire to be free, and my equally strong desire to be loved made it even more confusing. It would have seemed easier to submit to social pressures and conform. I guess I am not built that way. I did, however, like my peers and predecessors. I tried to have the best of both worlds by being free, but hiding that freedom from Anne wherever possible. It was evident that she did not want to deal with the truth. That seemed to hurt her and cause her to lash out at me. Because of her beliefs and what she had seen others do, she felt justified.

It made sense to me that if that were going to be the case, maybe we had better trust each other enough to see other people now before we got much older. We had been together since we were 14 years old. I knew that I would need to "sow my oats" before settling down.

Anne had a different idea of how life would progress between us. The way she saw things, I belonged to her and that had nothing to do with me doing anything with anyone else. All of a sudden, I was fighting the same battle that my parents had fought for so long. I wanted the security of love and constant sexual relations with her, but I wanted the freedom to find myself too. We had already shared some tough decisions about life together. That is what happens when kids, or even grown people have sex. Would I slip into a pattern of pain or have the courage to change?

WHO'S LOVING YOU?

...but since you came to town, I am spinning around with my head hanging down, and I wonder who's loving you?
The Jackson 5

I had been through quite a journey in self-discovery. What I was finding out about myself was very disturbing. Not many people really knew me. I never really felt like I belonged. While hanging on the block I was considered kind of like a punk but I got along with everyone. I would rarely if ever put up a fight when the other guys would pick on me or attempt to impose their will in any given situation. Starting a fight with me never really seemed worth it to them or me. I was always good at all sports so that was how I got a free pass through all of the gang wars and individual battles.

When I became a teenager, I was already in high school. I had to deal with too much shame on the block that I lived on because of the fighting that went on at my house and the frequent visits from the police. I had attempted to "kill" myself one time while in junior high by drinking ink from a couple of my pens. I had gotten in some trouble there, and I was drastically looking for some sympathy. Through the years I had obviously cried out for help. This kind of behavior was an indication of what would come later. I remember not feeling comfortable in my skin. I knew that I had the "potential" that everyone saw in me, but I had no idea how to realize it. I would have given every ounce of potential for a small piece of joy or happiness. That is what made drugs so attractive to me. It was a cry for help from the soul.

High school went relatively smoothly. I went to Forest Hills in a rich, white Jewish neighborhood. It was quite a coincidence that they were two-fare zones away too. This was becoming a trend. Most of the affluent white communities were. This time we had the option of taking the Q-6 and then the Q-60, or the E or F trains a couple of stops to 71st and Continental where we would then have to transfer to the G train and ride one stop to 67th Avenue. Then we would have to walk uphill two long blocks. There were no more of my boys the Smith brothers and many of my junior high school friends went to other high schools, but not my God brother Wayne. My mother was working behind the scenes all of the time trying to make sure that I was getting the best opportunities. I am sure that she and her best friend, Wayne's mother, Deliah, had a conversation about where Wayne and I would go to high school.

I cut a class or two, but I was a jock in high school. I started out that way, anyway. I played varsity baseball in my sophomore and junior years, but by the time I was a junior in high school, I was much more interested in hanging with Anne and the Trotters that I was in school or any extra-curricular activities. I knew I was pretty good at sports, but I did not have an image of myself actually playing in the major leagues or the NBA. There were plenty of guys that were better than I was, I thought. I did not have the confidence in myself to think that I could live that dream. It was soon to be made plain to me what was really possible in my life. I quit the baseball team in my senior year after spending two years being one of two black guys on our team. I played along with Stephen Gilliam, who started and played 1st base. He lived around the corner from my house and had come up in Jamaica Central Little League too. I got tired of going to practice just to sit on the bench in the games. That was something I was not used to, having been a starter and an all-star most of my life. So I quit, and the coach was pissed. His senior second baseman was graduating the year before and he was going to need me that year. I did not care. I was smoking pot daily and getting sex regularly, so I did not think that I would miss the varsity and I was pretty sure that they would not miss me.

I went to school with Ernie Grunfeld, a 6'4" forward on the varsity basketball team who was being groomed for college and the NBA. We were in the same boring hygiene class and missed it about the same amount of times. When graduation time rolled around, the hygiene teacher, who was one of the physical education staff, failed me and passed him in the class. That wasn't right. I took it as revenge for me not playing baseball that final year. That was their way of getting back at me. Even though I attended the graduation, something that my mother really was looking forward to being at, it was mainly because I was playing the baritone horn in the band that I was allowed to attend. Here I was graduating high school at the age of 16, yet I still had to deal with the possibility of not graduating or being able to participate in the ceremonies. That would have been devastating to my mother. She had put in a great deal of effort to get me to that point and would have been cheated if she could not have seen me walk down the aisle. There were many little incidents of racism, both hidden and overt that happened during my school years. I believe this was one of them. I spent that summer in summer school way out in Sheepshead Bay. I had to take the long train ride to a really hot school with no air conditioning. I had to do it to get my diploma and I had to have that. I participated in the ceremony, but I would pay for choosing not to play baseball that last year.

I graduated high school at 16 years old so my options were limited. I was tired of school and just wanted to be out of it, but I had no plan. So I did what any red blooded American kid would do. I went to college where I learned how to socialize. It was there that I started to think that I wanted to do radio or something in the area of communications. I also did what most of my friends were doing; I learned how to chase girls, play cards and shoot dope.

After all, even though I may have been smart enough scholastically to handle college, there were other life skills that I still needed to bone up on. For instance, I had to learn how to deal with that first real rejection from a woman and that was enough to make me say the two words that would haunt me for some time to come. Those two words were "fuck it" and it was what I would say to myself as a way of either hiding my feelings or as a way of not acknowledging that I even had feelings. After all, having feelings just made me more vulnerable and vulnerability was not a desirable trait in the world I was dealing in. Those two words, and that feeling of frustration that they epitomized, would be the one constant in my quickly changing world.

I started getting high because I really liked the way pot made me laugh. I enjoyed life so much better when I was able to look forward to the laughs I got from the euphoria that the marijuana created. It was when I got to college that I had my first real taste of rejection. A girl that I thought that I could really love, decided to break my heart. She was much more mature than I was and she already had a boyfriend, just like

I had a girlfriend. That kind of thing never really seemed to come into play when I felt drawn towards someone. I had scruples and would not mess around with the girlfriend of a friend or anything like that. I was drawn towards this young lady and was ultimately brokenhearted that she did not feel the same way about me. It was then that I felt the need to sedate the feeling of emotional pain with some heroin, even though I knew it had the potential to ruin lives. It was the drug that had changed the path of so many of my friends, changing them from mere observers of the war to participants, even seasoned veterans. This all happened to me before the age of 18 years old. "There are many rooms in my fathers mansion..."

ESCAPISM

...I was talking to a cat the other night; he said what
everybody' looking for today...escape-ism.
James Brown

It did not take too long for me to realize that I loved
heroin too much. No wonder people got strung out. I
was too smart for that, though. I was going to be the one
that did not get beat down by dope. It sure was a wonderful
feeling to be able to get high on heroin. The feeling was this
warm sense of well being that erased the pain from the years
of embarrassment and insecurities. It was a place where time
stood still and where cares and worry had no place. It felt like
a place that I could easily make my home.

The high was the reward for the chase it took to get it.
The excitement created by the adventure of getting the money,
finding the drugs, finding the "works", finding a place to "shoot
up," then being so cool about being high that no one would
know. That was an exciting adventure—in the beginning. It
was a weekend sport and I was a weekend warrior at first.

Then I found out that heroin would prolong and enhance
my sexual experience. Dope would help me to be the super lover
I always wanted to be. It is amazing how confident I became
when I knew that for the price of a bag of dope I could control
the bedroom action for hours! What a boost to my ego that
was. That made the drug a very necessary component of my

life. What a bonus it was to gain confidence, the adulation of women, and be able to lose my mind for how ever long I could stay high. Ever since I was a young kid, not having to think all of the time was a goal for me. As time went on, it became my priority to get high. I could stop whenever I wanted to, I told myself. I just didn't want to. Weekends turned into weeks, then months.

I had spent a year and a half, wasting time in college. I was 16 when I enrolled because I was too young to do anything else. I wanted to get away from home, but I was tired of school. I had no real vision of where I wanted to go or what I wanted to do. It was confusing to be so young and to have already lived so much. The drugs were starting to be the center of my life.

This really did not fit my image of myself, so I decided to join the Army to try to turn my life around. I figured that I could turn my life around by joining the army and going to school while serving. With my total disdain for authority, this was a big decision. I never would have submitted to that kind of discipline if I had not been truly desperate. So I joined with a buddy. It happened to be the buddy that had turned me on to my first shot of dope and with whom I was getting high with almost every day. It worked out o.k. for a little while. I was clean through basic training anyway. I got buffed and was in the best shape of my life. I was sent to Radar school in Ft Huachuca, Arizona, close to the Mexican border. In Mexico they had something called "Mexican mud," a very high-grade heroin. So once I was able to check that out my addiction continued there. No matter where you go, there you are.

After coming home on leave before going to Germany for my permanent party tour of duty, I was given a going away party. I had no intention of taking any drugs with me to Europe, but we smoked pot that night before we left. The pants that I had worn the night before at the party had an empty reefer bag and an empty pack of Bambu rolling paper in the pocket that I had forgotten about. They were empty except for some slight residue. It wasn't like I was a really big international traveler. I was really looking forward to growing up and doing something on my own. For the first time in a long time, it seemed like my parents, friends and family were proud of me. It looked like I was going to finally live up to some of the potential they all saw in me. That all changed in an instant the next day at the airport.

Of all the suitcases that were not searched, security randomly picked my bags to be closely scrutinized. They must have already known something was there. I can still see the agent opening the bag and going directly to the pants and the pocket, holding it high for all to see. The dogs must have sniffed it out. Could it really be true that I was getting busted for this, and now? That put a real damper on my arrival to Europe and my attempt to get my life together. Something always seemed to be getting in the way of me getting my life together and this was further confirmation that I just was not getting it right. I did not consider at the time that my drug use and my behavior were causing my troubles. No matter to what extent I went to try to get my life together, it was always going to be something I would have to overcome in order to do so.

The act of being detained on my arrival to Frankfurt, Germany made a terrible impression on my commanding officer. He, like many others who were in the Army at that time, was from the south and had been in the service since the 1950s. Here I was, a Negro from New York thinking that I was going to beat these "lifers" at their own game. That was not my attitude going in, but now I was in survival mode. I was out in the world for real and I was going to have to fend for myself. This was going to make a man out of me, one way or the other. It was a recipe for disaster.

When I finally made it to my base, I was offered an Article 15, which is a form of court martial. I had never been in trouble with the law, remarkably, while in the streets. Some New York survival skills kept me from admitting to anything. It did not seem right that I would get fined, busted down to an E-1 private, and lose the respect of those in charge over something like this. So I fought it and I was able to beat those and other subsequent charges while in the Army. I was very disappointed with the turn of events. So I got high. I later found out that there were no possibilities of getting the education that I was promised by the recruiter. The recruiter and the Army had outright lied to me about my chances to get an education while serving and I was determined to get justice. That is another time it is evident that God stepped in and saved me from myself.

With all the drugs that I was able to find in Germany it was just a matter of time before I ended up a military prison. I had a captain who was my immediate superior officer who took a liking to me. He could not understand why I was not in college somewhere playing basketball or baseball. He obviously had a lot more confidence in me than I did. No one else outside of my mother had actually shown such confidence in me.

Then, mysteriously, the Army came up with a new regulation that would allow enlisted drug users to be honorably discharged, thereby keeping one's coveted benefits. I had earned those benefits by virtue of making it through the very tough basic and intermediate training. It was as if they had created the Chapter 16 just for me. Moreover, it was as if I had wished it into being. The only other experience I had with creating something like that was when I was trying to figure out a way to get high. Magical things seemed to happen then too.

That was my way out of the Army and I took it. I had joined on the buddy program with a friend, Mike Scott, that I had been getting high with in my college days. He was in Germany with me, but I had to leave him there. He was later able to take advantage of the same loophole. I felt ashamed that I was going to be going against my word to him and my family, and even felt bad about not keeping my word to the Army. That was true even after I found out that they were jerking me around. I wanted to have integrity and be a man of my word. That is not how things would play out. That would not have been in my best interest at all.

Joining the army as a geographic cure for my fledging addiction was an act of desperation. The result was not what I expected or desired, but surely it quickened my awakening. The shame of coming home earlier than expected was quickly devoured by the frustration concerning the amount of energy I expended trying to be abstinent from drugs and attempting to be a productive member of society.

When I returned from Europe, I made attempts at college and lost a few good jobs. I was soon faced with the realization that I imagine many addicts face. There was the realization that I was mentally and physically addicted to heroin and cocaine, and those around me that were painfully aware that I had a problem. We were soon to know the depths to which I had sunk.

WHITE LINES

...ticket to ride the white line highway; tell all your friends, they can go my way. Pay your toll, sell your soul; pound for pound cost more than gold.
...Grandmaster Melle Mel

I had been stealing from friends and family to support my habit. Everyday was an adventure in creation. Everyday I had to come up with a way to get high. It was all that I could think of. Nothing else held the promise that getting high and leaving reality held. I was running from myself and could not get away fast enough. I had other aspirations and the foundation that my mother and father had given me had become a small and ever so quickly fading voice, lost in the windstorm of my life.

The fact is, I could not be trusted, nor could I trust myself with what seemed like the simplest of tasks. I did not have the self-discipline to do anything that had anything to do with money. As spoken prophetically by the character Pookie, played by Chris Rock in *New Jack City*, "That shit is callin' me, man." I tried everything I knew or heard to try to prove that I could control my drug use. I knew that it had become a problem in my life, but I did not want to let it go. Getting high is what I knew and was good at. I would make some futile attempts at suicide. They were as feeble as the ink-drinking incident back in Junior High School. It was an ugly fact that I would live for what seemed eternity. I would tell myself that it did not matter how low I sunk or what I stole because "this" time I would kill myself by an overdose. When death was not the result and I had to face the consequences of my actions, my shame created an even greater desire to die. It was then that I felt like a Prisoner of War. I was prisoner of war being tortured to give up information that I did not have. The question life was asking me was did I really want to have life more abundantly?

There would soon be a turning point in my life as a soldier in the war with drugs. If there were any past secrets about how low and foul I was living, it was now totally exposed and denial was no longer an option. The crisis came when I messed up some drug money. I was now selling drugs to support my own habit and like an addict is prone to do, I used all of the drugs I was supposed to sell for one of the most ruthless crime families in the neighborhood. It was not the first time I had screwed up a package, but this time I feared for my life. These guys had a reputation to protect and I was sure that they would not forfeit their credibility in the street just because they liked me. If there was any seed of doubt that they would do whatever was necessary in order to recoup their money, it was dispelled when they stepped to me and told me that they would beat me down for the money even though they did not want to. Embarrassingly enough, I had to go to my uncles to ask for money and protection. My mother's older brother David, and their sister's husband, also named David, came to my rescue. They covered my ass that time, but told my parents. I still tried to lie about it, but soon after I came to another event that proved to be a turning point in my life.

Feeling like the end was near for me, I went on another wicked run. By now I was so filled with shame and guilt, I would have welcomed the serenity and absolution of death. I had inflicted a great deal of pain on my loved ones. My arms looked like they had been the targets in a dart game. I was ridiculously bruised and visibly afflicted. At the time I was bringing home some high quality Columbian cocaine I would get from Union Street in Brooklyn.

My good friend and get-high buddy, Billy, was bringing home the top-notch heroin from Harlem. He was getting those drugs from the neighborhood where he worked as a funeral director at one of the most prestigious funeral home in New York. I was getting too high, so high I could touch the sky. It is a wonder that I did not kill myself after all.

Billy was more than just someone I got high with. We had a real connection with each other. He grew up on Inwood street like I did, his birthday was in October one year and four days before mine, and we both shared a love of good conversation, women and good drugs. We both were willing to go to great lengths to satisfy those desires. Billy and Michael Scott were the ones that I had first started shooting dope with back in 1974. The strain of maintaining drug buddy relationships was stressful enough to have caused us to not be seeing as much of Michael at this point in our addiction. After all, Billy and I were bringing home the drugs, so we did not see a reason to keep getting anyone who was not chipping in anything. Mostly we wanted to have more for ourselves.

One day while shooting up by myself in my room in the basement of my parents' home, my father slipped in and caught me. It was like a scene out of a movie, a really intense scene. You know, the one where the father says, "Show your mother your arms," and then the mother lets out a blood-curdling cry. Only God knows what she must have been feeling about all of the hope and promise that she had been holding on to for her son. To now see me as the same as all of the other dope fiend kids from the neighborhood was very painful for her. As far as she could see, I was dead to her. I remember it being the only time I saw my father cry. He must have felt the frustration of not only being unable to solve his own battle with alcohol, but also now seeing his son falling prey to the same kind of lethal enemy. I am sure that he was dying two deaths at once.

Getting busted by my father and the whole blood curdling scene that day in my house was the first time that I can remember having a real spiritual awakening. For the first time, I felt as if I was truly being myself, or at least being seen for who and what I was, even if part of who I was a greasy, sleazy dope fiend. It did not look very good. It was my first real taste of reality and it felt surprisingly good to have the covers finally pulled from over me so that I could be exposed. Denial was no longer possible or necessary. Something happened inside of me. I surrendered that day and decided to seek help. From that point I seemed to get a glimpse into the future. Though my father and mother sobbed in anticipation of their loss, I was able to tell my father in that moment that somehow I knew that everything was going to be all right. It was a strangely calm, yet incongruous feeling. That was my first real taste of blind faith.

***

Little did I know then that it would be among the last times spent with my father. A few days later as I was attempting to detoxify myself on the living room couch with quarts of Colt 45, my father came in and went back out with some people. They never came in and I did not know them from looking out the window. My father offered compassionately to bring me back some beer. I remember declining the offer saying I would be alright. That was the last time I saw him alive.

Later that night the police knocked on our door. It was about 2:30 AM when the flashing lights outside conjured up the fears that one lives with as the family of a police officer. You always suppress the subconscious thought that one-day they will come to the door to bring the news that we knew was always possible. When I opened the door and the policemen wanted to come in and begin a search for my father's weapon, my fears were confirmed before they spoke that truth. In the blink of an eye, he was gone.

You never know what it is like until you become the news story. It is one thing to watch the news and another to be it. Dad became a casualty of war when he was killed that night with his own gun. That happened when he probably caught one of his drinking buddies trying to steal his service revolver as he was coming out of a nod. They were in a dark little room above the launder mat on the boulevard on December 22nd, 1978, right before Christmas. I am sure it was not the first time that his revolver was stolen and held for ransom, so I guess Pops decided he was not having it this time.

The story is still somewhat convoluted. There were seven or eight people at the scene of the crime, but when they called 911, they told the paramedics that my father had had a heart attack. He had a heart condition that he was keeping very quiet about and there was very little blood from the wound. I think they must have cleaned him up, but I have not been privy to the grand jury investigation. My father, we would later find out, was carrying nitroglycerin pills on his person so that helped with the deception about how he died.

Why would I care about all of that? It would never bring my father back. I had already done the best that I could do to have someone that I trusted to go and get his body. Late the next day I got a call from a friend of the family. Miss Pecola had known both my mother and father since before they had met each other. She implored me to not believe everything that I had heard about the way things had gone down. I was skeptical, but intrigued, so I asked my friend, Billy Chambers, who was not only a great funeral director and mortician, but was also was one of the guys I was shooting dope with—to go to the boulevard and get my father's body. Billy and I had grown up together on Inwood street. We had developed a close relationship over the years that was made even closer by our mutual love for shooting heroin and cocaine. We had just had our first disagreement in the years of our friendship. We disagreed about some money owed by us to some of the drug suppliers we were using. Even though we were at odds that day, our love and respect for each other allowed us to overlook any negativity in this time of crisis.

He would make the discovery that the paramedics didn't bother to investigate. He found that my father had been shot in the neck and had either bled to death or had a heart attack after being shot. That set into motion a media frenzy that would end in the arrest and conviction of my father's murderer, George Adams. He was sentenced to only 3 to 7 years for the murder of an off duty police officer. In the streets there is a code that one has to live by. That code called for me to go out and at least find out who it was that had taken my father's life. Then it would be expected that I would exact my revenge somehow. I was not a killer, and it did not make sense to jeopardize my freedom and whatever ability I would have to take care of the family of which I was now the male head. I was angry that just when it seemed that I may be forced into having the courage to confront my fears about dealing with my father and myself, that was this tragedy that changed everything. It could not be about revenge, even when revenge would have been easily justified.

When I heard the leniency of the sentence for the convicted perpetrator of this senseless crime, I knew in my heart he had gotten off lightly because my father was a black man. Had this been one of "their own," a white cop, there would have been a lot more done about it. When it was a black man's death, there was always some kind of extenuating circumstance attached. This time the police, the emergency medical technicians, and the coroner's office really blew it. I often wonder and seriously doubt that we would have found the truth if Billy were not the one to make the gruesome discovery. The New York City medical examiner was Michael Baden. He has gone on to have an illustrious career. He has never been credited with bringing anyone back from the dead and this case was no different. That is the way it is in the hood. Shoot, that's the way it is in the world.

Dad was no chump, and was very loved by mostly everyone he served and knew. To this day when I meet someone who lived in the projects that he patrolled, I get nothing but stories of love and respect. My father was an intelligent and fair man. He had a problem with alcohol that he never solved in his lifetime. I believe that my youngest son is my father who has come back to this world. I often tell him that he had his turn now I am the daddy. That would now mean that in order to help his soul break the cycle of self-destruction, we would have to make some changes. I had no reason to believe that the life I was living at the time could possibly change into something that would change the generations to follow. I had to give it a try.

WHICH WAY IS UP?

...gotta get my direction together.
Richard Pryor

It was this turning point that helped me to fortify my decision to turn my life around at all cost. Now, I would have to get it right. I was 22 years old and it had seemed like I had done a lot of living in those twenty-two years. We decided that I would go away to a therapeutic community called Daytop Village. Well, it was more like an ultimatum. I wanted to get help, and I could not expect my mother to put up with my stuff. My mother was starting to find out about some of the things that I had stolen from her, like her fur coat and money. Those were the material things and though it hurt her that I would violate her trust in that way, mom was even more hurt by the way it seemed that her only son was turning out. I had even used my father's death as a reason to go on one last vicious run. Friends and family were especially vulnerable at the time of his death, during which time I begged for and stole money in his dead name. There was no bottom to the pit in which I was now not just falling in. I was diving in there. Deep down in my heart, and not so deep at that, I felt a great deal of shame and pain. It was not what I had planned or aspired to be in life. To the contrary, I had a lot of hope and promise for my life.

So now in order to get my life together, I would have to ask for and be ready to receive help. I would have to surrender in order to heal. To end up there was quite a journey. It was the hardest thing that I had to do up to that point in my life, and I did not know how difficult it would be. At least, once again, I would be doing something positive and moving closer towards being that I felt I was capable of being. That was the feeling that I had remembered having when my father actually busted me shooting dope and the charade was over. There was some of the relief of finally living the truth. The truth will set you free.

Daytop was like boot camp for addicts. They broke me down emotionally with confrontation, encounter groups and responsibility. It was tough going through the long, laborious process of helping to put me back together again. I really had very little options. There was not much that I could do to deal with the new responsibility of taking care of my mother and sister unless I got myself together.

During all of this, my childhood sweetheart Anne had been going through all of the ups and downs of my teenage and young adult life with me. She had endured all the trials and tribulations of my addictions and more. A part of my addiction was sex and the way I used it to find pleasure and control. As a young man, I had every intention of sharing love with whomever I could. It was the only thing that made me feel whole. Women in my life adored me and helped me to feel somewhat worthy of their love. I planned to make love to anyone that would have me. I tried to find ways to do that and still have the stability of a relationship with Anne.

The main benefit of having a solid relationship with her was consistent sex and companionship. I needed someone that would believe in me no matter what I did. Nanette's loyalty was unbelievable. At the time, I could not believe that she could possibly love me as much as she showed, and if she did, there must have been something wrong with her. That kind of love seemed to smother me and it scared me. I had seen what the two of us had in the relationship that my parents shared and I knew that would never work for me. Just the fact that I was young and wanted to sow my wild oats was reason enough to want to have the best of both worlds. Whenever the pain of not living up to Anne's expectations of a relationship became to great, I would always try to give her the option to bail out. She never took the option and stood by me through it all.

My freedom to do as I pleased was more important than the stability of a relationship, up until this point in my life. At this point I was reasonably certain that I could find sex, if not love without a problem. After the reality of addiction set in, I felt like I was damaged goods, so I was then very grateful to have my childhood sweetheart, or anyone that cared about me, still in my life.

With all that I was going through, it was good to have companionship. That kind of devotion deserved to be rewarded and I was going to give it a try. Most importantly, I was really trying to get my life together. So imagine my frustration with the goddess of destiny when six months into what was a very successful rehabilitation, I got my girlfriend pregnant. She had come to visit me upstate and we had a conjugal visit. I think it was before we were authorized to do so, but who can tell love when to bloom? It was the springtime when it happened, and we had not made love since the winter. As much as we were used to sex, that was a long time to be without. It is no wonder that without any kind of protection that we would run the risk of getting pregnant.

Here I was trying to get my life together and now I was

going to have to deal with this. We had already been through this scenario before, and had chosen to not allow the pregnancy to go full term. We were much younger then and this time I felt like she had paid her dues, so I made the decision to try to make it work. It was another turning point in my life.

Not long after finding out that she was pregnant, we found out that she was having twins. Here I was again. I was trying to do something positive in my life and yet I was still creating situations that seemed to be testing my resolve. I had to now try to figure a way to take care of my growing responsibilities with nothing to work with. My mother was willing to take my girlfriend in and allow her to live in the upstairs apartment of her two family home, but only if we were married. I did not know if I wanted to go that far. My girlfriend and I had been on-again, off-again for years and even though I felt like the stability might be good for me, I still had some reservations. It seemed that it was worth a chance. Nobody was ever going to love me more than Anne, and her loyalty was proven. I thought her to be sometimes very possessive about my love, but what did I have to lose? I was coming back from the jaws of hell so anything that happened had to be cooler than that, right? Maybe being married would make me more responsible and help keep me straight. Either way, with the children coming, we knew that we would be tied to each other for life.

Well, six and a half months later, two and a half months prematurely, I got a call while I was upstate. I was not slated to return to the city for good, or be done with this phase of the program for another eight to ten months. The call was to tell me that my girlfriend had gone into premature labor. I caught the morning van run into New York City, an almost three hour trip. I went directly to the Jamaica Hospital to find that the doctors there felt that the children would have a much better chance at survival if they were born in a hospital that was more experienced in the delivery of premature children. That meant that we would have to catch an ambulance ride from Jamaica hospital to New York hospital where their facility was qualified to handle what was a very serious situation.

After hours of very painful and scary labor, the doctors decided to bring the twins on into this world. It was a very exhilarating feeling to watch them both being wheeled out in incubators knowing that God had chosen me to be a participant in their creation. They were both weighing less than three pounds and one of them weighed barely more than two. Jason Troy weighed 2 pounds, 11 ounces. And Erin Vaughn weighed 2 pounds, 3 ounces.

When children are born, they usually lose weight before they start to gain some. I had sat with them for thirty hours straight as they fought for their lives in New York Hospitals neonatal unit. Both of them were small enough to fit into the palm of my hand. I know because I was allowed to hold them and talk to them in their incubators. The joy and amazement I experienced that day was tempered by my need to accept how tenuous the situation was. They were in need of oxygen and nutrition, but their tiny veins were too small in their bodies, so they had to hook up an IV to a vein in their heads.

After 30 hours of being by their sides and communicating what was going on to their mother, who had been taken to her own room, they finally talked me into going home. It was not long after that I got the call from the hospital that the more fragile Erin was not able to survive his thirty-sixth hour, it was very painful; yet somehow not a surprise. It was a miracle that Jason survived. My mother and Curtis tried to console me, but I was numb. In the course of one year I had lost a father and a son. Now I had to take this sad news to Anne and pray even harder for Jason to survive, and hopefully without deformity. I had named the stronger of the two with the name that their mother wanted most so that in the event of him being the only survivor, their mother would possibly find some solace.

New York Hospital was miraculous and God blessed Jason with continued life. I felt extremely guilty for having left them there to go home and get rest that night. I felt that someone made a mistake in their care, and that caused Erin's demise. I thought if I had remained vigilant about their care, as I had been doing, his death may have been averted. I quickly had to accept our reality and be strong. Anne was a very emotional person and I would need to console her now. To me somehow it seemed as if God was saying "One for you (God) and one for me." It was as if we had to make penance for the previous child that was aborted, but was still blessed with the opportunity to parent another. I also had to remember that I was still a resident of Daytop Village, trying to get my own life together. We somehow survived this drama and went on with life.

In Daytop Village, I had become something of a role model. When cornered, I seemed to have the ability to fight my way out. I seemed to be able to reach down within and say or do what was needed. The Daytop concept taught we could find no refuge, finally, from ourselves. It taught that until we were ready to confront change, and envision ourselves in the eyes and hearts of others, we would be alone. Daytop taught me to use behavior modification as a tool for change.

Daytop had a plethora of tools for teaching us how to do that, which included shaving heads, using signs and all kinds of disciplinary tools. Actually, it was a very scary place to be, especially at first.

When I arrived at the Swan Lake House in upstate New York, the residents were being put into a "tight house" where the lack of discipline amongst the residents is thoroughly addressed by the staff. At my initial interview, a staff member and a group of five residents lulled me, as the new resident, into a sense of comfortability. They got me relaxed with easy going questions about my past history. Then, all of a sudden, they blasted me with the reality about how much of a maggot I had been and why I had come to this place to change.

When I went through my interview, I did something you are not supposed to do. I jumped out of my seat when they verbally attacked me. I had begun crying when I was confronted about how I had done some really regrettable things. My back was to the wall, and the only thing that I could say came from the bottom of my heart. I told them that I knew I had done some really scummy things, but that all it was going to end right now. I sincerely wanted to heal so I surrendered.

Word spread about my seemingly unique reaction during the interview. Not unique because I was broken or repentant; because of the notoriety of the circumstances surrounding my father's murder, the media coverage must have reached Swan Lake. Knowing all that I had been through and the way I responded in the interview, the staff and my peers gave me a great deal of respect. All of that was further fueled by my apparent courage later that night when in front of the entire house of staff and residents I thanked the director—Tony Gelormino—for another shot at life and challenged the other residents to reexamine their reason for being there. All of that made me a respected member of the community immediately. That is not what I had planned, but I had every intention to live up to the image.

Months later on one summer day, one of our residents, Carl Timmerman, fell out of a canoe into the lake and drowned.

Nothing like that had ever happened at this or any other of the facilities. I believe that it happened later in the same day that my girlfriend and I had made love in the woods. It was the seed passionately delivered and received that day that would result in her pregnancy.

I had recently been through the media circus involved with the death of my father so I knew that I could be cool under pressure. It was that experience that helped me to at least be helpful during that incident.

So, six months later, when all of this happened with my children being born prematurely, my friends in Daytop and my family supported me. I was trying my best to change and to be responsible. After all, I was just one soldier in the war. I was expedited through the program in light of my situation. I decided that marriage would not be so bad and may very well provide the stability that my life would need in order to carry over the modest maturity I had acquired. It is one thing to stay clean while you are living in the protected environment of rural upstate New York. It is quite another to be back on the front line, hearing the sound of bullets flying overhead and wounded and dying all around. Temptation was waiting, but my resolve was bolstered by the expectations of my peers and the love and devotion to my new son. If he could make that kind of effort to be here on earth, I could do the same. I was determined he would not have to go through what I did. His father was going to be involved in his life a good bit more than my father was with me, and I was not going to have the problems with alcohol that my father had—so I thought.

When back in "the world," I settled in with my new, emotionally fragile wife, my barely five pound miracle of a son, my loving "Jewish" mother and my sister. I found work mostly with my mother's new "friend" Curtis McLain. I was happy to see my mother trying to enjoy her life. I know that they were concerned about how I would react to their relationship. All would be cool as long as he did not try to be authoritative and tell me what to do. After all, he was not my father.

Coming out of Daytop we were allowed to drink. My mother's friend was working as an electrician, but we also did cement and plumbing work as well. It was hard work, but it was an honest living. I was making enough to take care of my family and feeling pretty good about it. Although I had changed, I still had only modified my behavior. When I started to drink, it was only a small step for me to start smoking pot too. I could not tell anyone about that, but it made perfect sense to me. The problem was that it created a secret for me to have to live with.

The wives and family of people in rehab have the opportunity to support their family member by attending groups and getting information on how to "help" in the rehabilitation process. My wife and sister were involved. It gave my sister a forum for her own feelings and how she would deal with our past. She never did drugs like me but I am sure that she has had her own issues. Emotions have a way of manifesting themselves physically, as I would later find out for myself.

My new wife had issues too. Her way of using the information she would get from the experience would be to fulfill her needs for a secure relationship with me. By this time, my attitudes were starting to revert. I was still very interested in being a father, but not so interested in being a husband. A turning point was when after working hard for months in the heat of the summer mixing cement and busting bricks, I was able to support our family. I was giving my money to my wife like I thought a good husband would. When I came up short on my party money one-week day, I asked my wife to lend me some of my own money until I got paid that weekend. When she declined, I went ballistic. It seemed inconceivable that we could be a team if she was going to try to control me with my own money. It was then that I decided we were not going to make it together. I started acting like my father used to, and arguing like my parents did, and it really blew my mind. Here I was, back in the same house, doing the same things and getting the same results. I now know that to be the definition of insanity.

Soon it was out of control. My son was surely old enough to understand what was happening, or surely being affected by all of the fighting. I was seeing other woman and keeping more secrets. Somewhere along the line I met women that I felt compatible with and even fell in love with. Being married was a good excuse not to be able to get too involved with any other woman. As long as my emotions did not get involved, I figured I would be alright. My emotions did get involved sometimes and it was then that I started to feel like I was trapped in a really sick relationship. They say when two sick people are in the bed together it is a hospital, not a marriage. We were both very sick. We were both suffering from post-traumatic stress and did not know it. The whole thing was unbearable. I could not bear the thought of leaving my son, but the pain of staying was to great for all concerned. So I left. I moved in with a girlfriend who lived ten blocks away. That way I could still easily see my son, yet not have to deal with living in the house with my wife. So I thought. The situation seemed unbearable and I was angry. I thought I had a very good reason to say the two words that would continue to cause me pain—"Fuck it."

Not long after that, I built up some more secrets. It had been almost five years since I had graduated from Daytop and I was pretty detached from mostly everyone in the program. I started hanging around the people places and things that made up the old patterns I had lived. Destructive patterns that seemed more attractive, momentarily, than the pain I was feeling and the failure and disappointment I seemed to be experiencing. The next thing that I knew, I was shooting heroin and cocaine again. It happened just that fast. It was Thanksgiving and I was with my family at our annual gathering at aunt Vera's. I was with my cousin Debra who was a few years older than I. She had some dope and I knew where to get some coke. She had some "works" and I no longer cared or remembered how much pain and despair I had experienced before, and would probably get again if I used drugs. I had dismissed the promise I had made to myself and my dead father's spirit not to ever go back to that slavery of my spirit and my being. So I got high with her that day and it all spiraled downhill from there. It took me a few weeks of practicing controlled insanity by getting high only on occasion, before I was all out, full fledged strung out again.

I really wanted to die at this point. I felt that if I had to go through what I had already been through on the front lines of the war against drugs and addiction, I should die. My family history with alcohol, coupled with living in a place and time where outside forces seemed to be flooding my community with temptations that were stronger than I could resist, made me think I might as well just fall on a grenade. I knew very well that this time I was also risking contracting the AIDS virus, but there was seemingly no stopping my fate. It was winter of 1984 and I was feeling pretty bad. I was in and out of the house, stealing Christmas gifts from my family and selling them for drugs. I even stole the television my son had gotten. I sold the ring that used to belong to my father. A person who I thought were low live's were ashamed to be around me. It was either time to die or rise from the rubbish that my life had once again become.

Some things had been going right during this five-year period. I had applied to become an electrician, a job that would promise to provide a comfortable living for a person with my seemingly limited qualifications. By surviving a five-year apprenticeship at low pay, I would be qualified to make a lot of money, like $25-$30 an hour as a journeyman electrician. That sounded like a good plan. With the way things had gone in my life that was more money than I could hope to make doing anything that I felt I would be qualified for. So I jumped at the chance that Curtis made available by telling me when the applications would be given out. He let me know exactly what I would have to do to get one. There was a stringent application process, but I was willing and Curtis was very helpful. He had been around for a few years by this time and though he was no substitute for having my father, he certainly did his best to help. Curtis liked to drink a lot. I came to find out that most electricians did, and Curtis had been an electrician for quite some time by then. I liked to drink and make money while doing it, so I got on line and waited to get an application to become an IBEW Local #3 apprentice.

I waited four nights and three days for an application and the process lasted over six months. It was my best hope for the kind of life that I wanted to live. So when they denied me entrance into the program due to a "failed physical" I was devastated. I was in the best shape of my life being that I was "drug free," had been busting bricks and doing hard labor so I was in great physical condition. The only reason they could have possibly denied me was because I had been honest about my prior drug use. It was not as if I had a record or anything. I had been lucky to never have been arrested, just a few close calls. I just chose to be honest about my past because I had no intention on ever getting high again. You know, trying to do the right thing. Yeah right.

Well, when they denied me entrance into the program I could have just shot dope then and gave up. Instead I fought back. I wrote the union officials a letter. I told them that I had been looking forward to the opportunity to use the electrical profession as a way to provide for my family. I knew that I was in good shape and that nothing was physically wrong with me. I told them that if there were no more valid reason to deny my application, I would be willing to take my quest to the highest court. I had been among the first to experience integration in junior high and high school. I had been among the few Blacks in my school, army and other experiences. Now, I was trying to be among the first in a new wave of select few young Black apprentices. I was willing to fight for what seemed like my best chance for economic freedom.

In a couple of weeks I received a letter admitting me into the program. I am glad that as disappointed as I was about being rejected that I was able to be inspired to keep trying and not quit. Again, when my back was to the wall, seemingly, I came out swinging. I had nothing to lose and I prayed to God that he would work it out for me. I prayed that God knew my heart and saw the effort I was making to live in His light. I surrendered to whatever His/Her will for me was. It was another valuable lesson for the future. It also set the stage for me to be able to get the information that would truly give me the tools for a happy, joyous and free life. The opportunity to get that information would not happen before my fall from grace, but being in the Union would play an important part in my transition. Everything happens for a reason. There are no coincidences. Even when we do not know why we are doing the things we are doing, the Creator is guiding us. The willing heart will hear the call. The unwilling heart may have to take a fall. The plan is set for one and all.

The first couple of years as an apprentice went relatively well. I made it to work most of the time, and made it through school too. School was a requirement of being in the program. The wages were not that great compared to what we would make after we satisfied the 5 1/2 years of apprenticeship. Once I finished and became a journeyman, I would be making $25-$30 an hour for a 35 hour week. That was more than I had the chance of making on a job doing anything else I could think of.

So, you can imagine my devastation when I ended up shooting dope and coke again. I was in my second year of my apprenticeship and the attitudes I had developed in my previous 27 years of life were coming to the surface again. I was lost in the confusion of being married and wanting to be single. I began missing days of work, acting irresponsibly and jeopardizing the opportunity that I had fought to get. I was smart enough and aware enough to see that I was self destructing again. I had promised myself and the spirit of my dead father, that I would not let this happen to me, but here I was spinning out of control. In a lot of ways it seemed I did not have the courage to leave the responsibility of the roles of father, husband and son, but it seemed torturous trying to fulfill the roles. I was working with the tools that I had gleaned from the role models that were available to me, but my experiences seemed to not have prepared me for this. I was living the part of my life that was most painful to me, the arguing, fighting and misunderstanding. Society and my wife saw it one way, and I apparently was destined to see it and live it another way—my way. Using drugs was a way of forcing the issue. I knew that using drugs was the one thing that would cause everyone to abandon me. No one was going to want to live through that again with me. It was a well known fact that "once a dope fiend, always a dope fiend." The odds were slim that I would stay clean anyway. Being that I did not have the courage to leave, I would push myself out of the situation I was living in by being totally intolerable. The problem is that I loved my son with all of my heart and did not want to be away from him. It was a confusing and painful time and I felt like if this was the way life was going to be, then let me die—now.

When you get that low and feel the pain and desperation inherent in living through active addiction, it gets easier to surrender to something less painful. One day, after being on a vicious run of getting high, I wanted to go into a neighborhood church to pray to God for help, but even those doors were closed to me. I had done all of the terribly selfish things that dope and coke fiends do. At first I had promised myself that I would only sniff cocaine and heroin and that I could control it this time. When I started shooting both drugs again, "speedball" is what it's called, it was as if I had never stopped. I did all the things that I had done the last time I was using and more. I hid money in my socks, bought money orders, gave money to people I respected and told them that no matter what I said that they should not give it back to me until much later, only to harass them into giving it back, sometimes in the wee hours of the morning. I lied about where I was at and where I was going. I endangered my son by taking him to the places where I was buying drugs and I stole from him and the rest of my friends and family. The progression of my disease had advanced even when I was not using. The gorilla that God had minimized while I was not using had turned into an angry mammoth once I picked it up again.

I had angrily punctured myself in dozens of veins and had used myself like a pincushion in an attempt to anesthetize my pain. I was so disgusted that the church was closed because I thought that I could find God there. My life had had so much promise, but I was throwing it all away. I had not found a way to tap into the potential that my life was supposed to be. With the church doors closed, I ended up in a neighborhood funeral parlor, praying at the side of a casket of a person I did not know. It did not matter, I just wanted God's help, and at that moment I would have gone anywhere and done anything to find Her. Days later when I reached out for help, the director of the apprentice program for Local #3 IBEW, Buddy Jackson, was there for me. He arranged for me to go away to a 31-day rehabilitation program called Conifer Park. First he made me admit that I had a drug problem, and then he arranged for me to be picked up the next day and taken to upstate New York. Thank God. It is true that one must first die in order to live.

SURRENDER TO LIVE

I went to Conifer Park on January 29th, 1985. I had spent the night drinking wine and being depressed. Appropriately, there was a snowstorm happening in NY and I was staying at my Cousin Dolores' house. She and her husband Willie had put me up before. I did not want anyone else to see me like this again. The rehab was sending a ride to take me upstate to their facility in the morning, but I would have to find someplace to stay that cold and snowy night, while I prayed to be rescued the next day. Dolores and Willie lived in Coney Island and that was just far enough away from the SSJQ. I had taken that long train ride on the "F" train plenty of times before but never did I feel as low as I did that day. I was about a half step away from having to sleep on the train. Nobody will put up with an addict for too long, even one as charming as I was. With all the snow I wondered if the people who were supposed to come and get me would make the trip. I did not know if I would make it myself.

I was defeated and extremely angry. How could I, the role model poster boy for Daytop Village, and true war hero, be back here in hell? I had already beaten the odds by having gotten clean the first time. I wondered if I could do it again, and if so, would it become the junkie's nightmare where I would get alternatively clean and slimy until I died. My only experience with any kind of rehabilitation was a rigorous one and I was not looking forward to going through anything like it again. This was not rehab, though. It was something called recovery.

"In everyone's life, at some time, our inner fire goes out. It is then burst into flame by an encounter with another human being. We should all be thankful for those people who rekindle the inner spirit. "
-Albert Schweitzer

A counselor almost immediately recognized me. Ironically, he had been a staff member in Daytop. He remembered the respect and expectations afforded me. He asked me a question that made me know the immediacy of my situation. He made me know it was life and death by asking me "how much time did I spend in treatment before and how much time had it bought me in the street?" When I thought about it, I had spent about 18 months total in the program, and counting smoking pot, it had not bought me much time at all!! "Well", he said, "if you want to live you better get busy, because you only have thirty one days here." The clock was ticking. As in the past, I came out swinging, that is after a few days of feeling sorry for myself. I was told that the odds were that I would not stay clean. I was determined that I was going to be the "one in ten" that would get clean and stay clean. I was extremely angry at the world and myself for being in this predicament. Then I was told that I have a disease of addictions and that when I drink or drug or use mind or mood altering chemicals, it set off an allergic reaction to which I have no control. That made a great deal of sense to me and sort of explained how an intelligent person like myself could have been living the way that I was. That was something that I had never heard before, and it changed my life. In that moment I gained hope. I now was open to the information that was going to transform me as a person and make it possible for all the things that I have ever dreamed to manifest. At Conifer Park, I was introduced to the twelve steps and traditions of Alcoholics Anonymous and Narcotics Anonymous. What I was given to read about the program of recovery made sense to me, but it was the sharing that came from other recovering people that I was able to really identify with. People shared honestly about their experiences and many of their experiences were identical to what I had been through so it helped me to feel like I was in the right place. The people there gave me hope that I, too, could have life and have it more abundantly. There was hope that I would find peace and serenity in this lifetime.

I was given a statement that I would have to make every time that I spoke in a group setting of any kind. The statement was devised to remind me of my purpose during my time there, as well as when I left. The statement was and is indicative of a life lesson for me and I try not to forget it. The statement that I would have to recite every time I spoke and I would have to stand up and say, "I am Dr. Reggie and I am here to heal ALL of you!" When I said ALL of you, I had to wave my hand as if I was performing some kind of magic healing. Statements were what the staff created for almost every individual that came through treatment as a way of keeping us focused on what we needed to do in order to get what we needed.

Obviously, the guy, Carl, who had been a counselor at Daytop, remembered that I had spent a lot of energy and time into being a role model in the last program. It is a benefit of my personality that I will listen to the problems and situations of others, and often have feedback that others find usable. The harder thing it seemed would be for me to spend more time keeping the focus on myself. The lesson being—social acceptability does not equal recovery. It was then and there that I found out that I had a disease, and that it was a family disease for which I was not responsible for having. It was not my responsibility for getting the disease of alcoholism; but I was responsible for the choices I had made in activating and perpetuating the behavior surrounding my addiction. The things I had done while caught in the obsession and compulsion of active drug addiction would have consequences. If things were to be different in my life, my recovery would have to be my responsibility. I had had enough and I was ready to do whatever necessary in order to be healed.

I've learned that you can get by on charm for about fifteen minutes. After that, you'd better know something.

It was from this experience that I realized that I would not be able to drink, drug or use any mind or mood changing substances ever again, one day at a time. The way that it was made more palatable to me, and to all of the other addicts who had been used to using all day, every day, was to put in a shorter time frame. The very important lesson of taking recovery—and life in general—"one day at a time" was introduced to me then. It was an idea that had to grow into a lifestyle for me. It was something that I had to practice in order to make it my way of thinking and I had to do it if I wanted to survive, if I wanted to live. This was the real beginning of change for me and though I knew it was a "life and death" proposition, I did not know that it would get even more personal later on in life. And not much later, at that.

At the end of the thirty one days, it was time to go back into the war, back to the front lines, home to my neighborhood where I had been wounded. I had been healed and mended from the wounds that I had accumulated from the last battle. Now it was time to see if the information that I had begun to assimilate during my stay at Conifer Park had been internalized. Or would the old people, places and things be more powerful than my desire to live. I knew at a soul level, that a better life was available to me. I did not trust myself or my own thinking, and my past gave me good reason not to. Time would tell the story.

When I left to go to Conifer Park, I had decided that everyone and everything was dead to me. In other words, I was prepared to forget everyone for the sake of survival. When I returned, I had only one real attachment as far as I was concerned. I was only responsible and inextricably tied to my son, who was now five years old. Not only had he survived being born extremely prematurely, but he was doing very well despite the fact that his mother and I were not together and I had been living through some insanity.

Upon my return, I had to find a place to live. I asked a girlfriend named Jean, whom I had been seeing prior to my leaving to go to rehab, to help me find a place to live in Queens. I hoped that she would find me a place where I could live by myself for the first time in my life. I wanted a place where I could get my life together on my own terms. Jean and I had met on a ski retreat the previous winter and we had dated up until that time. We both had roommates staying with us on the retreat, so when we attracted each other into our respectively needy lives, it took some doing for us to create some private time together. In a moment of passion we made love that first night on the bearskin rug on the floor of the cabin. Then we continued to make love whenever and wherever we possibly could. I guess we were both very co-dependent at the time. I just wanted to be loved; was that so wrong?

So when I was in Conifer Park, Jean was my lifeline to the world. She was the only other person that I told where I was at. I did not think that it was anyone else's business. Besides, I had made promises to myself and others before. This time I was going to do it on my own, for myself and my son. So when it was time for me to leave and come back into civilization, I asked Jean to please see if she could find me a place to stay. Jean was not able to find a place that I could stay in, but strangely enough, she did find a place that we both could live in. I understood that to mean that even though she was willing to help me out, she had a different plan than I had. She had fallen in love with me and was creating a situation whereby she would gain her freedom from her parents. Jean had been through a lot and had ended up living in Astoria with her "Aunt." At least, that is the story that she told me, but Jean was very much the actress. She even aspired to be an actress. At the time though, all her performances were private. She was quite a performer, and I am not quite sure when she was being real or not. I satisfied a need in her and represented an opportunity for her to get away from her living situation and try to move in with me. I had never lived alone and I wanted to do something different in my attempt to get and stay clean. I just wanted to be free—free from the obsession and compulsion of drugs and anything else that could possibly trigger my addictions. I made it clear to Jean that I wanted to live alone but she told me that while looking for a place for me, she found a place for us. That was an opportunity to see if I was going to do the same thing I had done coming out of Daytop. I had gotten married back then in order to provide for my family—handle my responsibility. I was "in need" so when my mother said we could stay in the apartment if we were married, it did not seem like that much of a stretch. I knew that Anne and I had issues, but I thought I was smart enough and slick enough to give her what she needed and still be able to live my own life. Now, when I was coming home this time I was being faced with a similar decision. Would I take the easy way out by choosing to go for the okidoke, split the rent and move in with Jean?

I had a feeling that I should stick to what I knew to be the right thing, but once again, because I felt a sense of loyalty to someone other than myself, I chose to give living with Jean a try. Even though I could hardly save myself, I found myself trying to be a savior to Jean. They had just given me statements in the rehab that were designed to remind me that I need to keep the focus on myself. I am not here to heal everyone, but if everything went right It would work out for everyone. I was honest I thought. I told Jean I would not be able to live with her for long, because it was really important that I took the time to get my life together, and I could not see myself moving from the insanity of my marriage into another relationship. I needed to get to know myself. Jean said that she understood, but when it came time for me to leave, she decided to attempt a fake "suicide" by taking the contents of about ten bottles of Advil, or at least acting like she did.

I was very sorry to have to call her mother and tell her about what had happened. I had asked this young lady to keep my confidence by not telling my mother or anyone else where I had gone when I went to rehab. She had done that, allowing me the opportunity to just come back and grow up on my own before ever going back to see any of my family. It seemed unfair of me to do have to go against her wishes, but I had to go and I would have been more upset if she had done something more drastic and I did not tell anyone. It is the first time that the statement that I had to recite before anything I said to a group while at Conifer Park was applicable. I was not there to fix Jean, or even be responsible for healing her. The best I could do was save me first, the best way I knew how.

Though I felt like I owed it to her to support her as she had done me, it was like what happens when a person that only knows how to swim a little bit tries to save someone else who is drowning. They run the risk of being pulled in and drowning themselves. So I found a place living in the basement of some folks that I met at an AA meeting. They say that everything that we need is in the rooms of AA.

MAN IN THE MIRROR

I'm looking for the man in the mirror. I'm asking
him to make the change. No message could have
been any clearer...
Michael Jackson

I remember back in the day when we used to visit my aunt
on the holidays. My parents and their generation were
raised to eat everything on an animal. My godmother used
to say we would eat everything on a pig from the "rooter to the
tooter." She was right. I was one of the few people that liked
the smell of chittlins as much as I liked the taste. I looked
forward to New Years because I was sure to get some chittlins
and hog maws, black-eyed peas and rice, collard greens,
yams...man—please! That was some good eatin'.

On Thanksgiving my Aunt Vera, my father's only sister,
would cook all that and more. She could glaze the hell out of
a ham and hook up a macaroni and cheese that would make
you wanna smack your mama for the last spoonful! Is there
anything that we are more addicted to than the food we were
raised on? It was easier to see and want to quit the addiction
of drugs than it was to change my diet. Drugs are not socially
acceptable. People in our society revere a good steak, pork chop
or hamburger.

It is one thing to exhibit discipline around the use of
heroin or cocaine. But you get a lot of peer and family pressure

when you say that you don't want to eat any more meat. Your mother starts looking at you really funny. My mother began to think that you are trying to say that the way she raised you was not right.

By the time that I was ready to stop eating meat I knew that I was on the right path. God led me to this lifestyle change for a reason. Even greater change became available to me when another recovering addict introduced me to something he called the Path of Sound and Light. The program of recovery was working for me and had led me to a relationship with a Higher Power of my own understanding. Finally I had developed a sense that forgiveness was always available for me through the Creator. After all, here I was, clean and sober for a few years, living a radically different and wonderful kind of life. I had done some traveling and had begun to do some of the things that I had dreamed about doing. I had become a DJ and was playing at many of the functions in and out of the fellowship. I got a great deal of love and respect for the way I was playing both music and basketball with my new friends in the fellowships. I had given up the dream of playing professional sports, but it was fun to be playing at a pretty high level again. I was getting to know myself, too. This Path, he explained to me, seemed to be an extension of the recovery program. It would end up being the motivation for creating the discipline I needed in my life. The Path was not religious or dogmatic, but it satisfied my spirit and my intellect.

After coming into recovery I soon had to deal with the divorce and remarriage of my ex-wife Anne. That was not a real problem because I hoped that her remarriage would take her focus off of what I was doing. We both were dealing with the resentments that had helped to break us up in the first place. I hoped that her remarriage would bring some sanity to the way we would be able to deal with each other. Up until then, we were still dealing with the pain of separation. We seemed to be trying to exact a price for the investment we had both made in each other. We had been together since we were 14 years old. I was then 28, and there was no way to make that time redeemable. I just did not want anything to get in the way of my ability to have a relationship with my son.

I had tried to hang in there as long as possible, but my addiction and desire for freedom would not allow me to stay any longer. Not only that, it was déjà vu all over again. There I was living in the same house that my mother and father had so many fights. Now I was in the same house doing the same thing with my wife and son, knowing that it would be very possible that my son would suffer the same results that I had if something did not change. I could not have done that to him because I loved him too much. Actually, I loved and appreciated Nanette too much as well. Ultimately, we were who we were and that did not seem to be compatible with each other. I knew that I had exposed myself to dangers that she need not be exposed to; so breaking up was an act of love for the greater good. We had to negotiate the terms of the divorce in a hurry because she wanted to remarry. I was willing to keep it simple and sign the divorce papers so that she could get remarried. In exchange I wanted a very inexpensive child support arrangement. I was just getting my life together and had no doubt that I would take care of Jason, but I did not want to be legally liable and vulnerable to the emotional swings of his mother. I did not want to have anything to do with the legal system, especially when it came to dealing with my son. I did not find out until later that they were moving 3000 miles away to Los Angeles and taking the only person who really mattered to me with them. That last weekend before they were to move, weeks after she had been remarried, Anne supposedly had told Jason that he and I should enjoy the time we had left together before they moved because he may never see me again! Once I heard that, I kept him. There was plenty of drama after that one. I was determined to stand up for the love I feel for my son and to not let our relationship be like the one I had with my father. After the dust cleared, they were on their way to California and I was on my way to a special kind of hell. It was a hell that I was used to, but not while I was sober and clean. I was devastated that the love of my life was being taken away from me after all I had been through. Had I gotten clean for myself or would this be an acid test that they talk about in AA? I was in a lot of pain.

It was the day that I said goodbye to him that I had a spiritual awakening and revelation. While sitting on the toilet I saw behind the darkness of my closed eyelids a bright white and yellow light and became overwhelmed with a feeling of all encompassing love. Right after that I was driven to go to a meeting, so I went to a convention of Narcotics Anonymous. While I was there I met Phil Biscoglio while I was sitting on a couch trying to isolate myself and my feelings while in the midst of hundreds of recovering addicts willing and available to share my pain. I was in a great deal of pain about Jason leaving for California. He had been a great motivation for my recovery thus far. It was very painful to know that he was not going to be close enough for me to be an actively physical part of his life. Living through that gave me the chance to practice what I had learned in the program and to find out who I was going to stay clean for. We had been told that sooner or later it would not matter who we got clean for that we would need to decide to stay clean for ourselves. In time, I would learn to reflect on the fact that Jason's life was a miracle in and of itself. If not for the grace of God, Jason might not be with us in the land of the living at all. In order for me to survive the emotional devastation that I experienced with their moving to California, I had to come to terms with the idea that we are all God's children. I had to be grateful that we had had the time together that we had already shared. I needed to maintain my resolve to have a father and son relationship no matter what, and be not as concerned with where he was as I needed to be grateful that he was alive and available. So when I had that conversation with Phil, I was certainly open minded and willing to learn. I did not clearly see how I was going to survive the pain but I knew that God had not brought me through all that I had gone through just to leave me hanging. I was listening to hear how God was going to speak through others in order to make sense and give purpose to this new experience in my life. Phil and I had a three-hour conversation about life, recovery and a "Path" that he was on that he felt I might be interested in. I had long since stopped believing in coincidences and was intrigued by the information he was sharing with me. I saw our conversation as being one with God.

Phil talked about the possibility of being able to go within, and have what we call in the twelve steps programs "a conscious contact with God." He explained that it is possible for man, as the child of God, made in His image, to meditate and consciously still one's mind. By doing so, a person could actually travel what he explained as "that golden thread" back to the Creator. His logic and information was resonating all through my being. I was very receptive to this new information. It made sense to me that all I ever wanted to do was lose my mind. Even all of the sex and drugs I had indulged in during my life was an attempt to still my mind. Ever since I had been a child and realized the way of the world, my heart had grown somewhat cold and skeptical that I would ever find that escape back to that original love with God. It was entirely possible that my mind was getting in the way. After all, it is often said in AA that "it is our thinking that kept us drinking." The question that I asked myself about "recovery" was what is it that we were trying to recover? The answer that I came up with was that we were trying to recover our right relationship with the God of our understanding. I had made great strides towards moving closer to that relationship. How I would deal with this situation and this new information would afford me the chance to evolve even further.

***

As Phil explained the tenets of being on this path, I was somewhat intimidated by what it would take for me to be involved. The prerequisites for traveling this Path seemed entirely too disciplined for me. In order to test this Science of the Soul one would have to;

1) not use any mind or mood altering chemicals
2) be a lacto-vegetarian—no meat, eggs, or anything made with eggs
3) to live a moral life with no sex outside of marriage
4) meditation for at least 1/10th (2 1/2 hrs.) of each day!

***

The question I had to ask was what the most important thing in my life is. What is my life to be used for? Why had I been blessed and spared the fate so many other casualties of the ongoing war for survival and self-determination had already suffered? What was I going to do to be worthy of the "Purple Heart" and conditional release that I had been bestowed with?

I was going through a great deal of emotional pain, and clean this time, without the use of drugs or alcohol to deaden the pain. I was open to the idea of being able to leave this world. If I could do so whenever I wanted, without having to get high or commit suicide, I certainly would be open to how. It took a few months for me to finally make it to one of the meetings called Satsangs, where a group of people who were on this Path met and talked about what the gist of it really is. When I heard more, I realized that this spiritual enlightenment was more satisfying intellectually than any religion I had heard. Even with the stringent criteria, it seemed less dogmatic than what I perceived as the religious experience. It was as illuminating as the twelve step programs had been for me thus far and a natural progression of it. I made the psychic decision to walk that path, or should I say, I decided to stop resisting an undeniable pull towards it. I surrendered to my higher power on the strength of faith, hope and the desire for love.

That was an extremely important decision in my life. As the story was unfolding, it was a natural progression. I was beginning to see how my Higher Power was moving me in a very specific direction. I was starting to see how going through the battles of my life and surviving the war was beginning to manifest change in my life and those around me. It was also a wonderful preparation for what was to come. Oh yeah, there was surely more to come.

ME & MRS. JONES

...I don't know if it's wrong, but it's much too strong
to let go now.
Billy Paul

In the process of creating these changes in both of our lives,
Dionne became pregnant with our son whom we would
name Jarod. I had already turned my will and my life over
to the care of God as I understood Him. Being in the "high
risk" group for contracting the AIDS virus it made sense for
us both to get tested before we went any further. If we had
been thinking straight we would have been using condoms.
It is amazing how people can know that unprotected sex has
consequences, but we will often take the chance that those
consequences will somehow escape us? After all, I had shot
dope, so how could I not expect that it was possible that I had
contracted the disease? Actually, that was one of the things
that made me feel the most insane about using again. Having
another child was not in the program for me either. Dionne
said that she felt like because Jason had moved to California
and she could see how brokenhearted I was about not being
able to have him with me, she felt like this was going to be
her gift to me and my family. Strangely enough, I believed she
really thought that. So we got tested for the AIDS virus. Then
we waited.

In that period of time after taking the test until the

results came back I felt a certain sense of peace. It was a lot like the calm before the storm or what it must be like in the eye of the hurricane. I was somewhat resigned to my supposed fate. I was getting the same feeling that I had when my father had busted me shooting dope in the basement. It was as if I already knew what the results of the test would be. It was as if all of a sudden everything was moving in slow motion and I could see how I had gotten to this place. My track record had shown that God had never given me more than I could handle and that even though I was constantly trying to improve my life and the life of those around me, I always had to pay for whatever I did in life. So if I were going to have to reap what I had sown, I would still have to live and deal with it. I started realizing how blessed I had been and how I was constantly being given a choice as to which path I would choose. A very limited choice for sure. All choices boiled down to two—would I chose life or death? Would I choose love or fear?

Of course, I was very glad that Dionne had found out that her test came back negative. That meant that neither she, nor the child she was carrying for me would be affected. It meant that Dionne and our child would be alright. Thank God for that. No matter what my results were, that was the main thing that I wanted. Considering that if my test were positive and I could have no more children, then so be it, I would be satisfied with the hand I was being dealt. If my results were positive and I had contracted this disease that was strangely and grotesquely killing everyone that it touched, I would need to be more concerned about living long enough to see my children grow up. I did not want to have to suffer the way I had watched friends and family suffer through terrible conditions caused by opportunistic diseases they had become vulnerable to because of being exposed to HIV. By then it was a great deal of fear and not much understanding surrounding AIDS. People were very much afraid to be around those who had contracted the virus because they feared that it could be spread by touching an infected person, using their plates and dishes, or certainly by having sex with them. The stigma and prejudices that were attached to this disease seemed very real. If I were diagnosed positive, everything in my life, or what was left of it, would have to change. I had to be sat down for my results, and that is never a good sign. By then I had a strong inclination that day in April of 1987 would be the beginning of the end for my life. As I expected, or should I say feared, the test had come back and mine were POSITIVE. What else could I expect? I think I better let it go—it looks like another love TKO.

The health care worker that informed me of the results looked at me like she was prepared for me to fall apart. She seemed baffled by my numbness. The scenario was quite familiar to me by now. Every time I would attempt to make a major shift or change in my life for what I thought would be better—wham!! Something would happen that would try to blow me out of the water. It had happened so many times before. Even still, I was in a state of shock when I heard the words, "Your test came back positive." In the blink of an eye my entire life passed before my eyes and heart. I also felt my future crystallize. In 1987, a positive diagnosis was a death sentence, plain and simple. Very few people were surviving the disease. Those who managed to survive were not talking about being infected because they feared they would be ostracized by society. That was a very real possibility, even probability. There would be gossip, whispers and fear would cause some to change the way they dealt with the infected individual and their family. You could get fired from your job for mysterious reasons if it were discovered that you had the virus. People would make assumptions about how you had contracted the virus. Moral judgment was passed on infected people even in social groups that had to have a greater propensity of infected individuals, like that in the recovery community. Plenty of people who had shot drugs had unprotected sex and weakened immune systems due to the lifestyles inherent to addictive behavior.

For some reason I was not surprised. It was as if something in me already knew. It seemed that when I was shooting dope for the last times, I knew that I was walking down this road towards being infected. The image of a wounded soldier limping in to the friendly home camp dodging both enemy and friendly fire is the one I get when I think back to when I first went into treatment. There had been some indications that something may have been wrong with my blood. I was in denial that the signs were anything potentially fatal. If I had wanted to be paying closer attention to the signs I may have been tested sooner.

Earlier in that year I had been in the hospital briefly to have my prostate scraped after an episode of urinating blood. There are few things that had happened in my life that had scared me more than the night I went to the bathroom for what I thought would be a regular piss. It turned out that it would change the level of appreciation I would forever have for having just a regular urination. After leaving the 2230 club where I had been hanging out that night, I decided to hang out with a female friend. She lived nearby and I was driving, so we ended up at her house. Dionne says that she put a hex on me and that was the reason for what followed, but that is debatable. I used the bathroom at Phyllis' and the strangest thing occurred. Instead of urine, a stream of blood filled the commode taking the place of my urine. That scared the hell out of me but I had to be cool. I needed to get to an emergency room quick and only God knew what they were going to do to me when I got there. It turns out that they had to put a tube down my urethra and they would need to do it without anesthesia. That did not sound cool, but I was clean and sober and did not want to take any chances on setting off the compulsion and obsession to get high. I would rather take the chance of having a tube forced down my penis while I was awake, with nothing for the pain. That was preferable to the possibility of letting the monster go again. This was a chance to see how well prayer would really work. I must have said the serenity prayer a thousand times that night—and it worked!! By saying the serenity prayer repeatedly I was able to focus on the eye center that I was learning so much about and have a sort of out of body experience. I would need to be out of body for a while.

It was suggested that I have my prostate scraped and that I would need a hospital stay in order to do that. While in the hospital my doctor Jeffery Sandhaus acted very weird about my white blood cell count, but I did not consciously acknowledge the warning he was trying to give me. There was a great deal of hysteria surrounding HIV/AIDS. The doctor suggested that He do a spinal tap to check my bone marrow. I did not really make the connection at first and I guess it was not ethical for him to tell me then what my status was because that was not the reason for the blood test. It was all hush hush back then about anything that had to do with HIV/AIDS. It would be that way for many years. I imagine that he had a moral dilemma of sorts, looking back. There must have been something that registered subconsciously during that medical adventure because I was not surprised or devastated by this truth of my diagnosis now. I accepted my reality as if it were that of a third party—in a detached manner—somewhat aloof.

My whole life passed before my eyes, just like in the movies. Maybe being cool about what was happening was my defense mechanism kicking in again. I seem to have had the ability to keep my emotions in perspective and deal with situations as they are happening without losing my mind. I had exhibited it when my father was killed, and when my son had died after premature birth, when my friend drowned while we were in rehab, and at other times in my life. It is not that I don't feel, just that I have been able to have self-control and to rely on a higher power. Self control is the very thing that I lacked as a very young child, as exhibited by my many temper tantrums and crying fits when I could not get what I wanted, when I wanted it. I had been the same guy who as a kid cursed out teachers and showed a intense disdain for authority all of my life. Now I would have to really practice the things that I had learned in the recovery process. I would really have to practice and understand the principles of the twelve step programs that had already saved my life. Now I was really being tested and we would see if I could practice what I was preaching. I had already begun to receive some great blessings by living what I believed to be a program of recovery from drugs and alcohol, and I was willing to live through any of life's challenges using that same program as my guide. I made up my mind that using the program that had worked so well for me up to that point would be the way I would deal with life when it got really challenging. This situation certainly qualified as being a true test of that resolve. Would I fear death and use that fear as an excuse to go back to my old self-destructive ways or would I have a psychic change and use the twelve step program that had the tools to make it possible for me to survive and thrive through this devastating situation?

PRAYER FOR THE DYING SEAL

***

I had lots of friends that were already dead and dying from both addictions and AIDS. The common school of thought was that it would just be a matter of time before a person would suffer and die from either one or both of these diseases. So, it made no sense to me to start using drugs again. The craziest idea would be that if I am going to die—then I might as well get high. In reality, I had been clean long enough to have experienced the real joy of living clean. I knew that dying would be the easiest way out of active addiction, but I probably would not be that lucky. If I started using I would no doubt suffer rather than die. Anyway, I had already learned that I was powerless over my addiction and that my life had become unmanageable while I was using. While I was using, I lived to use and used to live. That is not how I wanted to spend what I thought could be my last days.

The fact that I was already living "one day at a time" was the perfect preparation for what I was going through now. The benefit came from a literal interpretation of the words and idea. Sure, there was some short-term and not-so-long-term planning. I wondered if I would be around to see my older children grow up, not to mention the child that my wife was soon to have. I would have to do whatever it took to be here for them, because it was my responsibility to do so. I prayed to God for continued protection for myself and my family. I decided not to tell anyone beside Dionne because it did not seem smart to expose myself to public scrutiny unnecessarily.

If nothing else, I have always felt a paternal responsibility to all of my children, natural and otherwise. Now was my chance to prove that I had integrity, and I would have to do it without fanfare. It would be just God and me. Of course Dionne was an important part of the experience too. She and I were the only people that I chose to share my truth with. I did not want to worry any one of the many people who loved me with something that they could ultimately not help me with at all. There were no cures available and treatments were experimental, so the best that I believed I could do was to change my lifestyle as much as needed in order to enhance my health. I HAD TO BE AN ACTIVE PARTICIPANT IN MY OWN SURVIVAL.

At this point it is important to say that I do not hold myself up as an example of how the recovery process does or does not work. Though millions of people have used twelve step programs as a tool, and it has been effective where all else had failed in the lives of many, the results of what will happen in a person's life because of the application is not guaranteed by me or anyone else that I know of. That program for life has been an integral part of my experience and so it is impossible to tell my story without referring to its influence in my life. I have written this book because I was compelled to. It is not my intent to act as a representative for anything or anyone other than myself. The considerable influence the twelve step programs have had on my life, and the part that it continues to play, is inescapable. Writing this book is a way of sharing what my experience has been so that others can possibly find some identification with those experiences. It has been revealed that through sharing our strength, hope and experiences, we have been able to evolve together. That is the real purpose for me writing this book. You may be able to decipher something out of what has happened to me in my life, and I may do the same from the honestly shared experiences of others. The God in me salutes the God in you. Having said that telling my story here is an exercise in faith, here is the best way that I can relate to you some of the things that have been part of my reality since that day in April of 1987.

People often say that nothing in their lives could have prepared them for a particular situation like this one, but everything that had happened to me in my life had prepared me for what I was going through at that moment. The question is whether or not I would be able to draw from the wealth of those experiences in this life and death situation. Earlier in my recovery from alcohol and drugs, I had felt compelled to be baptized and was not sure why. At that time I needed to answer the call of my spirit. That call was leading me towards a quest for a healthier spirit. I had often wondered what "recovery" really meant. You know, what is it that I was supposed to be trying to recover? If the disease that I have is threefold— mental, physical and spiritual, then is balance in these the things that which I am supposed to be trying to "recover"? Then in my even more urgent circumstance regarding my impending death, I would have to be practice being even more vigilant about my lifestyle than I had been thus far. It would have to be a three-pronged approach to maintaining balance, and the most important of the three would be the spiritual. I decided, or should I say, I was compelled and motivated to work even harder to recover something closer to my "original" relationship with a God of my understanding.

The twelve step program was an indispensable tool that God used to show me how to create an atmosphere to recover these things completely. It is no coincidence that the situations and circumstances of my life were mirroring the knowledge that I was being given. They say that God does not give us any more than we can handle. For some time after getting clean I was still practicing behavior that was not conducive to recovery. I still had some of the same attitudes I had grown up with. I did not want to go to work daily, and when I went I was rarely on time. I was grateful for my job but I spent a great deal of time focusing on being clean and sober and having fun with this new found freedom and zest for life. I had begun to learn how to love myself and I wanted to enjoy what I had considered to be life on borrowed time. As far as I could see, I could have been dead because of the lifestyle I was living. I did not seem to believe that life was for working yourself to death. Even though more often than not people lived their lives in this fashion I was not going to wait around until some time later in life to begin to realize what my priorities were. I still had to learn how to find some balance between making meetings and fellowshipping with other recovering people and taking care of my responsibilities. In other words, I still had to learn how to grow up. There was much more to learning how to live a productive life than just not using drugs.

My son Jason, who had been the source of my inspiration to live, was living in California with his mother. She and I would argue almost daily about just about anything. That was the nature of our relationship. It was made plain to me by my actions when dealing with her and the circumstances that grew from some of those actions, that as long as I was dealing with our resentments I could not get better. I was still practicing insane behavior and that that behavior was not conducive to the recovery of my mental, physical and spiritual wellness. The pain I felt from my actions which included saying and doing things dangerous to my serenity and sobriety caused me to reach out and begin to develop a closer relationship with a sponsor. A sponsor is a person who can help to guide the recovering person through the steps of the program. The steps of the program were being successful in making miraculous changes in the lives of people who traditionally had been lost to society during their active addiction. It was explained to me that even if I could stay clean without practicing these certain steps in my life, I would be much more peaceful and happier if I gave working the steps a try. My sponsor led me through the steps and helped guide me towards my true goal—peace and serenity. Love taught me who was the boss.

I had understood that the first step in the recovery process suggested that we admit that we were powerless over our addiction and that our lives had become unmanageable. That was evident to me in the rehabilitation process at Conifer Park. Since then it had been nothing short of a miracle how my life had changed. I had been through all kinds of personal test that had given me the opportunity to see what would happen if I attempted to practice this program to the best of my ability, and in every case, things worked out well when I chose to invite God in and practice the program. After a while I came to believe that a power greater than myself could restore me to sanity.

The third step suggests that we should "turn our will and life over to the care of God as we understood Him." The kind of unrest that I was feeling as a direct result of my behavior compelled me to have faith in the program as it was laid out, so I asked God to take control of my life and prayed for Her to allow me to be a vessel of Her word and an instrument of Her will. I now understand what is meant by the advice that we should be careful what we pray for, because we surely will get it. My prayer has been answered, but not in the way that I had envisioned.

YOU CAN'T HIDE LOVE

...so why not stop try to run and hide. You won't find
out if you never try.
Earth, Wind & Fire

***

After that, I felt like I needed to get baptized in
a church, so I did. I had no intention of getting
involved in the church. I had a need to demonstrate
my love for God and accept His love for me. I had spent some
time going to church as a child, and I still had way too many
questions about how and why the church did what it did. My
mother was raised as a Jehovah's Witness, though she never
tried to train us in that faith. I came to find out that my father
had shown no real propensity for the religious indoctrination
of his children; he had a lot to do with us not being raised as
Jehovah's Witnesses. I had questions with every religion. After
all, why is it that God would only bless those living at the time
of Jesus with the kind of proof that I was seeking? Is faith a
prerequisite for entrance into heaven? Seeking God is a part of
what getting high was for me. I was trying to find God deep
in the inner workings of my mind. I did not know that I was
doing that then, but my spirit did.

While taking a fearless and moral inventory of myself,
I realized that a great deal of my behavior was rooted in fear

and insecurity. One of the glaring needs that I had been trying to satisfy was the need for love. I shared my deep, dark and grimy past with someone who understood the process I was in, and how important it would be to not have these "secrets." The fear of being seen for who I really was began to diminish. By shedding light on the very things that I feared judgment about, being thoroughly honest about what I had done, I was blessed with a level of emotional and spiritual relief. The emotional relief was more evident, but the spiritual relief allowed the universe to know that I was ready for what was to come. It also opened the way for the law of attraction, that spiritual principle that speaks to our innate ability to draw to us what we desire and are prepared for, to go to work.

I became willing to have God remove all my defects of character and asked Him to remove all my shortcomings. Then I made a list of all the persons I had harmed in my life so that I could later go about the business of clearing the wreckage of my past. Later in the process, seeking to make amends with those I had harmed and done things that I thought were wrong would be the only way to build a strong foundation on which to build the rest of my life. After making the list, I was amazed at how often I was given the opportunity to make those amends with people that I had put on the list. Some of them I had to go a bit out of my way to ask for their forgiveness, but for the most part there seemed to be something mystical about the way the people I was identifying as deserving amends would appear in my life again, and be receptive to my efforts. Resentments made it very hard for me to see where I had to ask for forgiveness at all!! I had to have faith in the process, I was told. I had nothing to lose. Among those I needed to forgive, including myself, I put my ex-wife Anne at the very top of that list. I did not want to forgive or be forgiven by her, but I had faith in the program. I had had enough evidence already to let me know that the program would work, as long as I worked it to the best of my ability, as outlined.

So the next step was to continue to take personal inventory—and when wrong promptly admit it. This was so that I could maintain a sense of sobriety and grow on the foundation that I was building. I would understand more better, through prayer and meditation, how I could have a conscious contact with God, as I understood Him, praying only for knowledge of His will for me and the power to carry that out. Even that would become clearer to me as I learned about the Path towards enlightenment to which I would be led. The Path would create desire for meditation and help me develop the kind of discipline that would be necessary for me to battle for life with this new disease I had been diagnosed with. I often wondered if I would have been as motivated to commit to a discipline so different from the behavior that I had learned to practice from childhood. Would I have been as willing to sacrifice so much of who I had been if I had not been diagnosed with AIDS? I am glad that I found out about and had a great desire to be on this Path before I was diagnosed. It was of great comfort to me to know that I wanted Him before I thought there was a greater chance I would be dying sooner than I wanted if I did not change. I did not want my seeking God to be a "foxhole" type of prayer activity. I had no problem, though, asking God to lead me in the right direction and praying that living the tenets of the path would be sufficient to cause God to spare my life. As it turns out, living as a vegetarian, practicing monogamy and meditation, as well as staying clean, would be actions that I am sure have increased the quality of my life.

As usual, those around me were seeing more potential in

my life than I could see in myself. I can't say that my esteem was low, but I did not envision myself with the kind of promise for success that others were telling and showing me that they saw. I was very grateful for the blessings that God had bestowed on me thus far even though I sometimes questioned the method with which some of life's lessons were presented to me. His grace and mercy seems to be without borders. I do know that I feel passionate about these blessings. I pray that passion will flow whenever I am given the opportunity to share my strength, hope and experience with either a group or an individual. Now that I was not altering my mind with chemicals I could feel God working through me and I knew that I had no real choice but to take the ride.

It was with this foundation that I had the faith to bare my soul and tell God and another human being the kind of person that I had been. I had to trust that sharing these secrets would relieve me of the guilt and shame that I was still experiencing. At least then I could clean out the wreckage of my past and begin to change. It is then that the re-circuiting or re-channeling of the energy that was stuck in a feedback loop operating in my mind began. That mindset and the patterns it created caused grooves that developed in my mind keeping me from a greater evolutionary pace. A psychic change was necessary for me to continue to attenuate my spirit.

Once I experienced the relief of sharing my "secrets," and realized that it was possible for me to face my fears, I was able to move on through the next actions that would further enhance my changing. I had to make a list of all the persons that I had harmed, including myself, and make amends to them except when to do so would injure them or others. That could have been a scary proposition and one that I might have skipped, but I had already had the positive experience of having the courage to challenge my fears. I had seen benefits of having faith in the process of recovery. Doing that had worked for so many before me, and I now had the strong desire to feel the joy and peace that I had had glimpses of earlier in my life. More of that was virtually promised to be the outcome if I continued to pursue further action.

So I ended up making the list and then going to the people on the list. After prayer, meditation and consultation, I believed I could ask anyone of the people on he list for forgiveness without causing any harm to them or me. For me that meant going to the people that I had begged and stole money from to get the drugs that I had craved for so long. The incidents that I felt most shamed about were the times that I had asked people for money during the drama surrounding my father's death. It was a time that I knew people would be sympathetic of my situation and be more willing to lend me money that I had no intention of paying back, and I took advantage of that. After I did those things I really felt pathetic. There seemed to be no absolving myself for doing such a thing, and it was one of the things that I really needed to make amends for if I hoped to grow spiritually and experience any kind of real joy.

SHINING STAR

...shining star for you to see, what you life can truly
be.
Earth, Wind & Fire

Since I have been clean and sober, I have greater joy,
peace, serenity and gratitude in my life. I am not always
living a balanced life, but in order to try to stay in
harmony with the forces of the universe I continue to take a
personal inventory—and when I am wrong, I try to remember
to promptly admit it. That helps me to keep a check on my
attitude and practice some measure of humility, and is another
suggested step in the recovery process. My attitude is among
the most important thing for me to keep in check. My attitude
and my thinking are at the core of my actions. Everything
begins with a thought. Everything that is was created by
thought. The holy trinity can also be explained as "thought,
word and deed." It is what we think that controls the way we
heal—or don't. Every cell in our body is "of God," in fact, IS
GOD. It has been said that man was created in God's image.
How we communicate our thoughts and feelings to the things
in creation seems to be an extremely important part of the
healing process. What we tell our cells and how we present
ourselves to all things in existence, is directly responsible for
what we create.

The information that I have been getting speaks to our

ability as human beings, and as "children of God," to have a true conscious contact with God. That means that I could finally have what I had been seeking all my life. There was a chance for validation that there is a God living inside me. Moreover, the Father and I are one. I mean, I had begun to have more faith and a much better relationship and understanding of our Creator. My relationship with God had grown as a direct result of being more conscious of a higher power in my life. That understanding that had come from the application of knowledge was fine—but I want to experience God in a super conscious state. Why super consciousness, you might ask? Super consciousness is merely a word or a meaningless term that sounds wonderful, and without a true grasp of what it means or the concept it represents, it remains merely a concept. Super consciousness represents expanded mind and it represents the flow of mankind into godhood. It is knowingness and an innate feeling that attunes itself to life. There is a super-intelligence that is everything that is. It is in everything from the molecules that make up what we have come to understand as being the building blocks of life, integral to the cycle of birth, life, death and regeneration. Super consciousness is life; it is God. The information that I have been blessed with leads me to understand that through prayer and meditation and by the creating of an atmosphere for both, it is possible for us as human beings to achieve a conscious contact with God. I am now and have always, as it seems, been seeking just that, even when I did not know it or could not identify it.

As a young child, I was pained by what I learned of the world. It was my great intention to change the world into a better place filled with more love and equality. I felt frustration and dismay at knowing that the world and the systems that run it are designed to oppress the masses. It seemed that I was powerless to change the world. That was a frightening realization. It caused me to want to die or live unconsciously.

There were two acts that gave me the feeling of death, ascension or at least seemed to still my mind if only for a moment. Those two acts were when I was having an orgasm and getting high. I realize looking back that those were the times that, for a fleeting moment, my mind seemed to be momentarily still. It was then that I experienced moments of super consciousness. It is in these moments that my egoic mind is shut down and union or the awareness of the union between soul and God is then possible. That probably is a big part of the attraction for humans to be addictive. My desire is to go beyond the mire of our limited thought, and experience that innate oneness with the original creative force, while knowingly having that communion with God, and not having to question whether or not the experience was real.

Now back in the day, that is not the conclusion that I had come to about my insatiable urges to get high and have sex. Then it seemed like fun and an escape from reality. After a while of doing both it became more work, and with it came a sense of being controlled by my own desires. I had become a slave to my own desires. The work it took to get high, and the integrity I had to give away in order to do so, became very frustrating. I was constantly chasing the ecstasy of the first time I had a sexual climax or had gotten high. I enjoyed the fantastic adventure of space travel. That is what I experienced with each time I tried a new drug or had a new woman.

Women were certainly massaging my ego by responding very favorably to our sexual experiences, as evidenced by their desire to continually engage. I have always been eager to please. That seemed to be a blessing and a curse. Just like the drugs, the women had selfish motives and they both would turn on me in the end. Somehow, competition between my desire for drugs and my need for personal freedom would prove to be a problem for most women. My need for freedom provided a challenge for women because society dictated that committed relationships are monogamous and I did not want to limit my opportunities for love. It seems that women enjoy a man that is concerned with pleasing them. Women would ultimately go to great lengths to maintain some semblance of control over me, and I fed into that behavior due to my need to be loved. It has had to be very frustrating for those people in my life that have relied on me fitting into a particular mold in order for their happiness to be achieved. I never want to be boxed in like that. It is too much unrealistic pressure being responsible for the happiness of another human being.

LOVE TO LOVE YOU BABY
Donna Summer

Even the act of sex and having an orgasm had begun to lose some of its allure after finding out that I had been diagnosed HIV positive. I was now "tainted" goods and had the potential to be a negative part of someone else's life by infecting them. I did not want that then and still do not. It has affected my self worth. I still enjoy sex a great deal, but I enjoy love and romance as much. I practice safer sex by using condoms but the idea that I could even remotely contribute to the demise of another human being is troublesome and restrictive. Concern over what could possibly happen to those I would have sex with for the rest of my life continues to weigh on my mind. It still does at times and has affected my relationship with my wife. At first the effect was because I did not want to risk her being infected. Later I began to wonder if I should leave home in order to protect her. I was constantly preparing all of the family for my eventual demise or departure, without actually saying that was what I was doing. It began to help me to deal with the emotional confusion when I began to more fully accept my reality and do some of the work needed for emotional healing.

I also had become bored with knowing exactly what to expect during sex. No matter what was done during the act of sex, the end was always pretty much the same. Ultimately there would be a climax that would last only momentarily.

During sex, the mind would shut down very briefly and in that moment I would not have to be concerned with the things of this world, and would sometimes get a glimpse of higher planes. I questioned the sexual act and wondered if there could be more to it or a way to prolong the visions, escape and experience. It is very gratifying to give great pleasure and love to another, and my ego looks for opportunities to do so. A very large part of me loves to love. We humans seem to be challenged to balance these feelings and how we share them with each other.

Getting "high" was the other time when my mind would shut down for a brief moment. The chemical reaction I experienced from the use of drugs and alcohol seemed to quiet the noise that constantly reminded me that I was not at peace with the world or at peace with myself. Those two acts, I came to understand, created feelings and states of mind that are attainable through prayer and meditation. It can be done in a wakeful state, thereby creating the kind of knowing and experience with love most humans live for. Having the discipline to practice the meditation necessary to achieve that state of mind takes consistent practice. Becoming willing to prepare the human vessel by not eating meat, and living a moral life so as to create the atmosphere for evolution to a higher vibration, takes great effort. The motivation of a life-threatening illness, or the pain and suffering of life itself, can prove to be factors that motivate us towards success in these areas. That has been the case in my life, and it has changed me. Even motivation that is based in fear can be changed or transmuted into being a love-based motivation. For a period of time after getting clean and sober, fear of life as it was when I was using was my main motivation for staying clean. As time went on I have had the great blessing of having that fear of getting high change into the love of being clean and sober. That love now remains the driving force in my life. I like who I am and what God has done in my life.

All of these things that I have been learning have had a purpose. All of my experiences have been leading me to where I am today and preparing me to deal with the reality that I have created. I understand that it is necessary to have a level of faith in things unseen, but it is important that I do the best I can to participate in my own survival. Cleaning the human body and preparing our earthly vessel for the fulfillment of our individual and collective purpose is one of the things we can do to participate. The effort to be made ready to receive and accept God's will for my life could very well be a lifetime endeavor. I find the effort to be well worth it. The destination called heaven is enticing, but the journey through this life has been filled with joy and pain. Whatever the case, I enjoy watching the adventure of life unfold.

IT'S A LOVE THING

...every time that you are near it becomes so clear—I
knew deep in my heart, it was love from the start.
The Whispers

In talking to people and listening to the way we humans
interact, it is evident to me that a major factor for the
spread of HIV is the simple desire of people to be loved.
That is part of the insidious nature of the HIV virus and of life
itself. Both are perpetuated by the need for love. To have access
to and enjoy more than one sexual partner and to be desired
sexually by others is the underlying reason for the spread of
AIDS. At the very least, people often do not want to limit
their opportunities for sex, and thereby love, no matter what
is said publicly. It is perceived that identifying oneself as an
HIV carrier would seriously diminish one's chances for sexual
partners. So in many cases people that may be infected do not
get tested so that they can continue to behave irresponsibly
without the guilt that direct knowledge of their actions'
consequences would present. Some that have knowledge of
their positive status find it difficult to share their status with
others for fear of the stigma involved with being identified as
HIV positive. Sex is the way that we often validate our love.
Sex is the way we justify our "lovability." In our society, sex
and love have been inextricably linked to the point that for
many there is little or no discernment between the two.

As humans, our desire for intimacy is real to us and should be satisfied even if our need for love is an illusion. The love we seek is within and always available to us, so we always possess the very thing that we seek. What we think we have to do in order to have love has been greatly perverted for the sake of commercialism. Our innate desire has been co-opted and used for the control of the masses. We are constantly being distracted and diverted from the love within, and instead we are constantly bombarded with images and other kinds of external sensory stimulation. That is not to say that there is not a place for lust in the grand scheme. From a different perspective, we would do well to remember that God is love. The Father and I are one. There is no separation between God and I. Therefore, I am love. As written in *A Course in Miracles*, "Healing, then, is a way of approaching knowledge by thinking in accordance with the laws of God, and recognizing their universality." "Seek ye first the kingdom of heaven, because that is where the laws of God operate truly." "When you heal, which is what we want, we are remembering the laws of God and forgetting the laws of ego." As mentioned in the bible,"the kingdom of heaven is within."

The way we create in this physical realm can be better understood by understanding energy. Learning about the chakra system is a great way to learn about our human relationship with energy. In yoga, chakras are associated with any one of the centers of spiritual power in the body. Each chakra is associated with a different human system like the endocrine, reproductive and so on. Becoming aware of the effect of energy on our bodies is important knowledge in enhancing our ability to heal.

It has given me a new perspective of sex and the way that it can be used to help enhance my ability to "know" I am healed.

It has helped me to see that sex has always been an exchange of energy. The act of sexual intercourse is the creation process for a reason. It makes sense that the way necessary for creation to perpetuate itself would feel so good and be so attractive. It feels great to create energy that is instigated in part by the friction in our genitals because that is the way that the energy ascends our being through our chakras. (See the chart and notes at the end of the book for more information).

From the first chakra, the genitalia and the reproductive organs, the energy moves up until it reaches our crown chakra, above the third eye or the frontal lobe area. When we have an orgasm, it opens up the pathway to higher realms, accessing God by energizing the "golden Chord" connecting our physical existence to that of the Holy Spirit. The Holy Spirit is in the part of the mind that lies between the ego and the spirit, mediating between them always in favor of the spirit. Orgasm, then, is the moment when we are truly God. It is when we have the ability to co-create and when we access the power that is Him. It happens so quickly, and feels so good, that we become addicted to the feeling and experience. I know I did. That, evidentially, is how I have been experiencing the sexual experience. I know that I am not alone.

Healing this, and any other disease, then, should entail a new perspective with which we look at sex and the need for love. To put them in a different relation will allow the motivation needed to stem the proliferation of the virus. "Human nature" supposedly leads us to sometimes lie to others and ourselves in order to get sex and love. If we begin to learn to be honest about who we are, moreover, learn who we really are in relation to God and the manifestation of that energetic life force, I believe we would be more motivated to experience sex in some new and excitingly purposeful ways.

I have begun to explore the science of Tantric sex as a way of harnessing sexual energy for the purpose of creation. I believed that I have explored a number of sexual experiences, but they had become mundane and repetitive, always with the orgasm being the defining goal. I believe that if we were to promote a better understanding of Tantric sex, massage and the concept that there is possible healing in the harnessing of that energy, we may begin to change our behavior in this regard. If men thought that each time we ejaculated we were moving closer to physical death, or at least, diminishing our human potential, maybe we would begin to have the conversation about how to change our sexual experience. Our addiction to the feeling of satisfaction is at the root of any change that is possible.

Though many in my life have loved me, I am still learning how to love myself more fully. A part of that education is my applying one of the great teachings of my life. That is learning to have the courage to be more honest about who I am without hurting others or myself in the process. As I share more honestly about who I am, and live more consistently with that reality, I have been magnetizing great information with which to make more informed decisions. It is a life-changing experience. It has been the motivation for using my life as a way of sharing hope with whoever may draw inspiration from it. Now that I am being more public about what my experience has been medically, I am getting a great deal of love and sharing from others who are in the same situation as I am. Many people have found the courage to share with me the particular situations that their living with the HIV virus has created. Some have shared what it has been like to have loved ones who have either died or continue to live in spite of being diagnosed HIV positive. I have recently shared my story with people only to find that they too are HIV positive and that some even have spouses that are HIV negative, like my wife. The term for that type of couple is serodiscordant.

I am getting more feedback from others who are surviving long term with a disease we were told would kill us for sure. We all seem to concur on one thing. The mind is an extremely powerful tool that can be your best friend, or your most formidable foe. Extraordinarily, the choice is ours. On a daily basis, even on a minute-by-minute basis, we have the power to change our thinking to something that serves the universe and us in a more evolutionary fashion. We have the ability to choose. That is what makes us different and having a dominant adventure here on earth. We have all knowledge available to us in our minds. We all possess skills and gifts that we have forgotten how to use. It is said that we use a minute percentage of our minds, and I agree. Our evolution is centered on our ability and desire to remember what we already know. I am that I am and that which I am is moving to remember.

Most of us are unconscious and oblivious to our evolution. Our minds often seem to perceive change, and all of the external factors that contribute to change, as a threat. When our minds react to change in a defensive way, we are further entwining ourselves in a number of reactions. There are emotional, chemical, spiritual, physical and mental repercussions to resisting change. The body is an intricate maze of systems that keep our souls functioning on this plane. The mind is the master controller of the body. There are functions of the body that we do not control or have to think of maintaining. The heart beats and we breathe without having to think about it at all. Those functions are motivated and maintained by the part of the mind that is above our consciousness.

Every cell in our bodies is a universe in and of itself. Serenity is directly proportionate to the level of acceptance that we are able to experience. The body seems to respond well to being in serene places. The attitude of serenity is a choice that works towards the healing from within.

REASONS

...the reasons that we're here. The reason our feelings
won't disappear.
Earth, Wind & Fire

Our emotions have been proven to have a great effect on the way our cells respond to the demands of the mind. Stress is the result of our mental response to our emotions and the amount of stress that we are affected by is relatively controllable. We have to make some decisions in maintaining a healthy atmosphere, an environment for healing. The serenity prayer has been instrumental in assisting me to know when to surrender my ego and acknowledge that external factors are determining my reality. When I am conscious and aware that I am fighting to prove that I am right, not wrong, when I am justifying behavior that is self serving or just not doing the things that will serve me, it is time for me to surrender to heal.

I am grateful to have had the opportunity to travel the world. My attitude about life has been influenced by the knowledge that I have a couple of diseases that, if left untreated, can be fatal. The way we experience life begins with the mind. My mind told me that it made no sense to "wait" to live. My mind told me that given the opportunity to live, I want most passionately, to be FREE. Freedom is not something that someone can bestow or deny. Freedom is a state of being—

a state of no mind. There are people who have been imprisoned who have attained a much greater degree of freedom than those who are walking the street. Shackles can come in all kinds of things. Nelson Mandela had to have achieved freedom in his mind and heart long before it manifested as his release.

Our desires have the greatest potential to imprison us, and those who would sell us the solutions, like the social consciousness seen in the media and other images, have created many of those desires. Most people are slaves to their own desires. The things that we want or feel we have to have kept us riding on a wheel of self-obsession. We often dismiss the universal principles that our human experience is designed to teach. Though I value my physical freedom, I am looking to enhance my mental and spiritual freedom.

In my travels I have been a student of human behavior. I have sat at the feet of yogis in India, and been taught enlightenment by masters in the east and west. I have practiced a program that has led to the recovery of my mind, my physical well being, and the balancing of my spirit, to the best of my ability. In 1989, soon after taking initiation in a yogic practice, I went to India to meet my guru. I had been intrigued with the answers that I had gotten to many of the questions that I had about the Path and the great wealth of knowledge I was getting during my investigation of it. The answers helped satisfy me mentally about many of the inconsistencies of religion.

At that time, I had developed a different kind of understanding about God. That understanding had evolved by my experience with life, but more relevantly, my experience with 12-step programs had begun to shape my relationship with a God of my understanding. God loves, and in effect, is love first and foremost. God is also non-denominational and is the unifying force of this universe and beyond.

I have learned to practice greater and greater amounts of faith, believing in things unseen, and have had more and more personal opportunities to see how universal principles work. When I practiced the principles of the recovery programs, I consistently and continually reaped the rewards of favorable outcomes. This further emboldens my faith. It also made me hungrier for a personal understanding of the 11th step, which states that we are able to have a "conscious contact with a God of our understanding."

That desire was born from the thought that such a thing is possible. The desire created a magnetic response that drew that opportunities to get that knowledge to me. Attitude and the way we respond to life has everything to do with the way our individual stories unfold. I was motivated, once again, by pain.

I was in my third year of recovery when I was faced with the divorce of my first wife and their imminent move to California with my eight-year-old son. Jason's mother and I had gone through so much, including constant arguing over the amount of time we were able to spend together. I love my son very much and he had been the largest part of my foundation and my desire to live through my fight with addictions. Now, his mother was taking him 3000 miles away and I was powerless to stop her from doing so.

At the time, we had not yet settled anything regarding that move and how it would affect my relationship with my son. My ex-wife's apparent disregard for me born out of resentment and anger was evident in the message she gave Jason before he came for the weekend of what would have been his last visit before moving. Somehow, Jason had leaked it out so that it got back to me that his mother had said that he should enjoy his visit with me because it would probably be his last. Now, we decided there would be joint custody with no restrictions and very little forced child support. It went down like that because she and her boyfriend had already decided to get married, so they were a little anxious for her divorce. I took advantage of the situation so as to not make myself vulnerable to the whims of either Jason's mother or the legal system. I had no doubt that I would live up to my responsibility as a father, but I was happy to at least not have to worry about a large child support payment. That proved especially important when my work situation became erratic. I was less susceptible to the emotional outburst I had seen women are prone to. So we settled and they got married.

It seemed strange and vindictive that out of all the churches in the world, they decided to get married in the one right behind where I was living at the time. Now, she was talking about taking him to California. Her attitude about maternal rights being more important than mine, and the trouble I was having seeing him when I wanted with him living only a few miles away, I knew that I would have to take a stand right then. I decided to keep Jason with me until we were able to hash things out in court. That did not go over to well with Jason's mother and her new husband because they were planning to leave New York that Monday. Pandemonium was the result. That Sunday, when it was time for him to go home, I called to tell her of my decision. We argued and I am sure that she felt that her being the mother would prevail. I was living with Dionne and her two children in an apartment above Gloria Jackson's dance studio on Merrick Boulevard. It was the dance studio that I had danced at years before. It was where Savion Glover was learning to dance and within walking distance of the homes of James Brown, L.L Cool J, NBA star Mark Jackson, Russell Simmons and many others. That day, it was the place where all hell would break loose.

She came to the house with her new husband and others. I anticipated them coming, so I called the police and a couple of my friends. When Anne, her new husband and their crew got there, they began to bang on the door demanding that we send my son out. We were defiant and called the police again about the disturbance. When the police arrived, they were two female cops. I could not believe it when they sent two female officers out on a domestic dispute. They automatically took her side and demanded that we open the door and send out my son. I feared that if I did not get a more reasonable circumstance that I would lose my son for good, so rather than open the door, we called 911 again so that they would send out more cops, hopefully some men!

By this time they were frantic outside our door. His mother was screaming how I was a junkie putting her son at risk. She was saying whatever she could to get her way and to reinforce her faulty belief that the mother has more rights than any father. The female police officers were banging the door in trying to intimidate me to succumb to their pressure. I decided I had to take a stand for this because I believed my position to have merit. After all, I had joint custody, had been clean for a few years, did not have any legal situation in place for the new circumstances and deserved a chance to work that out in court. That was not how it was going to go down if I opened that door.

Most of all, I wanted my son to know that I would fight for the right to be with him.

The male officers, including a captain, finally arrived. I let them in and contrary to the claims that my ex-wife was dramatically screaming about our inability to be parents, the cops could see we were clean and my paperwork was in order. I had joint custody and there was no imminent danger, so we would have to go to court to settle it. I thought she would have a heart attack at that point. There was total disbelief on her part and all those with her. We had kind of played what if game around certain situations, and in all of them she held the idea that she was mother and that would rule. This new reality seemed incomprehensible to her. Too bad. That is how it was going to go down. I had taken a stand for something that I really believed in, in the face of possible catastrophe and it seemed to go my way for the moment.

The victory was that my son, though nervous about leaking the information that caused this particular conflict, now knew that no matter where he was, I would fight to see him if need be. They soon left for California after we went to court to settle what the new visitation arrangements would be. That was a very painful day, the day that I had to say goodbye to my son. I felt pain for the perceived loss of the opportunity to have the kind of relationship with my son that I had not had with my father. I had already forged an extremely strong bond with Jason and I wanted the chance to play ball with him and watch him grow. That was going to be much more of a challenge with him 3000 miles away. I had a great deal of anger for my lack of control of the situation, because there was nothing that I could do to change things. Then there was some level of fear about who I would be without the motivation of being a parent. Jason had been a major part of my wanting to get and stay clean and contemplation of changing my entire life made me at least wonder if I would revert back into old behavior patterns that had proven to not serve me very well in the long run. After all, with Jason gone, maybe now was the time for me to try to go it alone. Without the need for me to provide a healthy atmosphere for my son, it seemed like it may be the time for me to try living alone for the first time in my life.

The major lesson would be for me to understand that after all that Jason and I had been through together in his young life, with him being born 2 1/2 months prematurely, weighing only 2lbs.11ozs. and having a twin brother Erin who did not survive because his even lower birth weight and underdeveloped organs, it was important to remember we had already survived much. The lesson was that it was not as important "where" Jason was. The blessing was "that" he was. It was tough on all of us having survived the tumultuous relationship between his mother and I, but our ongoing need to inflict further pain on each other even after our separation and divorce further proved our inability to extract ourselves fully from the pattern of arguing. It was a pattern that satisfied a sick need that had developed as a symptom of the posttraumatic stress we had created from our personal time at war. It hurt me deeply to consider living life without my son, but this was another lesson in surrendering. I would have to learn how to surrender to my powerlessness over the situation about their moving to California, just like I had to surrender to the Creator by acknowledging my disease of addictions. At best, I would grow emotionally by applying the principles I had been learning in recovery. I had been told that there would be a time when I would be tested to see if I really wanted to stay clean and live. I watched as many others had been tested in similar ways. Some had experienced greater and lesser tragedies with mixed results. Faith is believing in things unseen. This was my opportunity to have faith in what had learned in the program of recovery. That would mean getting past my emotions and learning to live a day at a time. A day at a time is basically all we have anyway. This was another chance to realize that I would have to surrender to heal.

OH MARY DON'T YOU WEEP

Tell Martha not to moan.... cause Pharaoh's army
drowned in the Red Sea. Oh Mary don't you weep—
tell Martha not to moan.
Take 6

That day, I did something uncharacteristic. I went in the
bathroom and I cried tears of despair. During those
tears of resignation and inside the self-preservation of
surrender, I was moved. I needed to get away and take a ride
somewhere to clear my head. It so happened that there was an
NA convention being held in upstate New York that weekend,
so I went. Pain was the motivation. I was seeking relief. The
suggestions of the program had worked thus far, so I followed
another one by making a meeting and being around other
recovering people to help me deal with what I was feeling.

It was there that I met Phil Biscoglio. The meeting was
so synchronistic; it had to be spirit led. We sat and talked
for hours on a couch in the middle of hundreds of addicts.
Somehow we had been drawn to each other and Phil had gone
on to tell me some of the intriguing philosophies about the
Path of Sound and Light. He explained the concept of there
being a golden thread that connected the Higher Power and
us. He explained just enough about the philosophy to pique
my curiosity, especially when he told me that people who were
initiated onto this particular path would have the benefit of

only having to live a maximum four more incarnations before our souls' eternal return to be at home with the Father. What I was going through made me more receptive to the idea that I could be working towards going "home" to be with the Father. I wanted to learn more about this science of the soul.

I was glad to learn that there were many books and a living guide that would teach us the way to escape this region of mind and illusion. That concept resonated within my heart. I had a desire to still my mind and leave this world behind, finishing my work here once and for all. So, after much further investigation satisfied my mental and spiritual curiosity, especially the non-denominational, non-judgmental nature of the path and the eastern philosophy, I sought initiation and was glad to receive it in April of 1988, one month after finding out that I was diagnosed HIV positive.

The promise of what traditional religion considers being salvation and the assured release of my soul from the cycle of life and rebirth helped to anchor my faith. It made it easier for me to deal with the additionally life-threatening diagnosis of HIV/AIDS. I had already applied for initiation before being diagnosed. Now, the tenets of the path seemed even more logical. It was becoming more evident that an unseen force was guiding my life. At the very least, I was being given choices that many others seemingly were not being exposed to. It would be my choice to surrender and make the changes necessary to participate in my own survival, hence my evolution, or to be subjected to the consequences of something different.

There were some criteria to effectively experimenting with this lifestyle. The tenets of this path are strict vegetarianism, meaning not eating anything with meat or eggs in it. That seemed like it was going to be really hard, especially when I began to realize everything that is made with eggs or egg whites. Changing my diet would prove to be quite a challenge. I learned not to eat anything with a face or a heartbeat. The intention behind daily meditation (1/10 of the day= 2 1/2 hours), a clean moral life including no sex outside of marriage and no drugs or alcohol, is to create an atmosphere for spiritual growth and the discipline to do it. Now, where I came up, in the SSJQ, we did not eat like that. Our parents where born and raised in the south where they cooked and ate everything to survive. I learned how to do the same. I grew up eating everything on an animal. We used to say that we ate everything from the rooter to the tooter. That included chitlins, pig's feet, hog maws, ox tails, ham and everything else. We ate it unconscious of what it meant to either our own bodies or that of the animal. All I knew is that it tasted good. When it was explained to me that we are what we eat, and that the animals were the highest form of life besides us humans, I began to see some light. Then it was further explained that the meat not only slows down our vibratory rate, our mental ability and that meat potentially makes us sick. The digestive process, it was explained, would hinder our ability to engage in the experiment of meditation as a tool for ascension and enlightenment. I always wanted to have more discipline in my life but instead I ended up not having very much discipline at all. This was going to be another step in the process for me to gain even more discipline that was needed to not use drugs and alcohol. It was coming at just the right time because having been diagnosed with HIV meant changing my lifestyle if I was going to have any hope of survival. Being on this path was sure to be a challenge, but a good challenge and a great step towards healing.

From getting high to sex, I had always been looking for a way out. Now I was being offered another clean and sober way to live. If I could practice anything close to perfect adherence to this relatively extreme discipline, I was promised to have life and have it more abundantly. Anything short of perfection was still good. I had always admired the Muslims and 5 Per center's when we were growing up. They were a sect of the Muslim faith that practiced discipline and focused on knowledge of higher ideals. At the time it seemed dogmatic and hard, so it was not easy or fun enough for me to practice it.

The Path came in my life at the right time. I was motivated at first by pain and later by fear of dying. I imagined dying without having fully lived and having to come back over and over again until I got it right and learned the lessons my soul is destined to learn.

Soon after Jason left for California with his new family, I found out I had a life threatening illness that was decimating our community and the world. I knew my soul needed saving. This Path would prove not only to be the promise of salvation and of having a guide through the afterlife; it was another step in my resurrection from the war of this life. By not eating meat, and not being the indiscriminant sexual partner that I had been previously, I was buying time that others in my similar situation were not being blessed with. I had surrendered to this Path and my Higher Power, and the process was healing me.

GET AWAY JORDAN

I'm going cross the Jordan to see my Lord.
Take 6

In 1989, I visited India to meet my guru and teacher, Maharaj Charan Singh Ji, and spend time at the place where others from all over the world gathered in peace to sit at the feet of the Master. It was quite a trip beyond what my mind could have conceived. It was very exciting to think that an old dope fiend like me was traveling to this exotic far off country in quest of greater spiritual knowledge. I flew through London to Delhi, 18 hours in the air. There was a full day of travel from New York to New Delhi, with the stopover in London. The trip to Beas, India, a small city in Northern India, on the border of Pakistan, would be an eight-hour train ride from New Delhi. That part of the trip would come the next day after an eventful night in the hospitality of those in Delhi graciously available to receive those of us making the trip.

It was a culture totally opposite from the one I had experienced here in the west, but I was open minded and ready to experience the adventure. I had made up my mind that work would not be the death of me and that I would only work as much as needed to be responsible for my self and family. I had spent unemployment money to get to India, but it seemed so synchchronistic and mystical that I had to go. What would be more worthy of life and money than to seek one's spiritual fulfillment? Friends and my new family questioned my plans, but as was my practice, I did my own thing and went alone.

There was a real war going on in India when I made my visit there. There was, as is now, a misunderstanding about whose land is whose. It was strange to see military personal patrolling around with Russian made rifles. I took comfort that there were many people who had made the trip from the US and other places in the world. A clear and efficient system had been put into place for those of us drawn to see our Guru in person. I arrived at night and followed my explicit instructions to take a taxi to the place where I would stay the night before catching a train the next day for the agonizingly arduous 8 hours north to Beas. I had no idea what to expect, so when I got in the taxi that I had paid for at the station, I did so on the faith that God did not bring me to India to kill me. That was the attitude I had and I had to laugh to myself as the taxi sped through the dark streets of Delhi. We had no headlights to show the way, but neither did any of the other speeding cars that overpopulated the streets that night. There seemed like there were way too many cars going way too fast, on a much too dark road in this strange and foreign land. I just laughed and treated it like I was on a rollercoaster or something. We arrived at what was an army fort safely. We were greeted by a strict, but courteous gentleman at the gate. The gate was opened after careful inspection of my passport. After further conversation with the taxi driver, and being questioned by the guard, I determined that the taxi driver was trying to get paid again for his services. Here was something that I was used to, somebody trying to rip me off. Some things are universal I guess. The guard was weary of both our stories, obviously, because though he dismissed me and had me taken to the bed made available for me to sleep in until the morning, he kept my passport. My last international trip this far out of the United States had a disastrous start as well. I had not expected what had happened, and I wondered if this trip would hold the same type of surprise. After that adventure in Germany I figured anything was possible in my life. I did not know what was truly going on, but I knew that I was powerless, so I surrendered to the will of God and this guard. I was apprehensive and very tired so I had no trouble going to sleep and deciding that I would find out my plight in the morning.

As it turned out, the same gentleman who had dealt with the situation the night before had come to return my passport. He did not say much, but this morning he was adorned in regal military attire that indicated he was an officer of some high rank. I was then much more impressed with his level of humility. He was a fitting representative of the Path and very unlike what I would expect from an authoritative figure such as he. Besides waking up to the conclusion of this adventure, I was culturally shocked by the city of Delhi. I was to awaken to the sound of strange music blaring from the temple through the streets of Delhi. It was like I was in a movie or a documentary or something. The music was a non-stop chanting that filled the air with the aura of spirituality. Everything had been worked out about my wild and crazy taxi trip the previous night. Soon five of us all from different parts of the western world took the long slow train ride from Delhi to Beas. On the way we saw just how poor and different most of the country seemed to be. We had to wait more than once for cows to clear the tracks so that we could continue our journey. The train was extremely crowded in the economy class, and though our accommodations were somewhat better, this part of the trip was much more grueling. It had a lot to do with the constant smell of burning diesel from the train's smoke stack, the burning garbage along the countryside, and the constant stop and go for the entire trip. I doubt that we ever went more than 60 miles per hour for any longer than ten to twenty minutes at a time. It was surreal to say the least, but I was on my way to further enlightenment and that excited me for sure.

My roommate in Dera, the name of the complex where Maharaj Charan Sing Ji was living, was a young man named Joshua Samson. He was from The Hague, in the Netherlands, and he had been on trips to Dera before and had been there on this trip a few days before my arrival. Joshua has become a dear friend for life. He had parents and friends who were initiated into the Path, so he had much more experience with the Path than I. We stayed in the same "room" while there at Dera and often were chided by others in rooms near ours for making too much noise. The fact is we did a great deal of uncontrolled laughing about the things we shared. We were somewhat irreverent, yet respectful. It was quite an experience to finally meet my Master. My skepticism with religion and humans as an authority was something I had put to the side. I took the trip based on my intuition and the information I had learned from written information and Satsangs—meetings with other followers—that I had attended. While I was there visiting the center in India, I had plenty of opportunities to get close to Maharaji and ultimately to have a personal audience with him. He always talked about the importance of meditation and the creating of the atmosphere for meditation. That was the gist of his encouragement to his disciples. What I liked about the path is that it left room for any religion one chooses to follow. The intent of the path is to give more meaning to whatever religion or spiritual literature, like the Bible or the Quran, that a religion was built around. The path was geared to give greater understanding of all religious ideology. The path left room for the questions that my western Baptist sensibilities would create. As open-minded as I considered myself to be, I was still leery about going to hell like our western religions promised if I followed a path other than that outlined in the Bible. It was good to know that at least the path was more inclusive. I know that it was a great blessing to have been pulled to make the trip to meet him. I am glad that I responded to the pull to go. It was an educational and enlightening adventure. A few months after my return from India, Maharaj Charan Singh Ji decided to leave the mortal plane. He left us with a successor to teach us, but it was wonderful to meet the physical spirit that had officiated over many initiations, including my own. Through proxy he had initiated many others and me, it was still under his tutelage that we were guided. Energetically, he would always be at the eye center, our third eye, waiting to guide our spirits home. Gurinder Singh Ji would be available to answer our questions regarding spirituality and to be accessible through meditation. I continue to practice that meditation and follow that path to the best of my ability. I practice meditation nowhere near as well as I can, but as long as I have life I can get better. It has certainly made me a better Christian and given me a clearer understanding of what is related about Christ in the Bible.

I have been exposed to some of the cutting edge treatments for the treatment of the diseases I have been diagnosed as having. I was among the first to try low dose alpha interferon as a treatment for AIDS. There was a time in 1989 when it was diagnosed that I had only four T-cells fighting off infection. By definition that meant that I had full blown AIDS and by experience and later the opinion of my doctor, that meant I possibly had less than six months to live. Many others in my same situation had died horrible deaths from the opportunistic infections that living with such a low defense against infection had made them vulnerable to killer infections. AIDS, we had learned, is not the killer at all. It is the weakening of our immune system and the infections that develop because of our inability to fight them off is the killer. My inclination has been to stay away from the toxic medicines like AZT that were being offered and to rely on more natural methods like exercise, positive thinking, meditation, herbs and vegetarian food. I tried to be the very best father, husband, son, brother and friend that I could be and to be of service to the God of my understanding. I promised God that if He would have mercy on my soul and allow me to have life and have it more abundantly, that I would serve him. I prayed that my life would be used as a vessel of His word and an instrument of His will. I was afraid that I would not get to live very long and that seemed like such an injustice considering that I was finally a productive member of society. I was learning to be the person that I always wanted to be and felt like there was hope for me to be a part of the shift needed in the paradigm. I was stepping into the role of a reluctant Messiah and saw more clearly how my life experiences could be shared and used to help others to do the same. I prayed to God for His will to be done. These things have all served me well. Through God's Grace and the company that I keep, the lifestyle that I have evolved into has allowed me to spend a great deal of "quality" time with those of you among the living. As far as I am concerned, all the time that I have an opportunity to get closer to the God of my understanding, is "quality" time. These are a few of my motivations for life. I pray that you have found your motivations for living, or at the very least, are hearing that small still voice that is that spirit that gives us life. That voice, if not further muffled, will whisper the things that you need to hear in order to create your own personal freedom. We muffle that voice with our own self-will run riot. The paradox is that it is when we surrender to our higher power is when we gain access to unlimited power.

We basically know the things that we are now doing that do not serve us well, but we often continue to do them, citing lack of willpower as our defense. I can't tell you how many people have told me after learning that I was a vegetarian, " I know I should stop eating meat too, but I just have got to have my meat!" More often than not, this would be coming from someone who is overweight, diabetic, or HIV positive. Even when sharing that I believed that vegetarianism was a contributing factor to the blessing of good health, with people who knew we were both positive, there was an unwillingness to change that (and other) aspect of their behavior. Smoking and drinking fall into the category of things that are important to find some discipline about. I do not claim to have the only way or the right way. I am simply sharing what my experience has been. Inherently our spirits will tell us what is right or wrong for us. I think a part of me does not want to talk about how disciplined I have been able to be for fear that it will send me into a spiritual relapse, that somehow by saying and claiming what I have been, will somehow jinx it. That feedback is still deeply embedded in my mind. Even after this long period of time living this lifestyle I feel somehow vulnerable to relapse. By writing this, I am purging that fear and further exhibiting my faith in God. I acknowledge this compelling need to share this information as a way of further allowing the still small voice to be heard.

I pray that this book will create a dialogue that will allow more people to gain greater personal freedom. I am gaining greater freedom by being able to share my strength, hope and whatever wisdom I have accrued from these experiences. It is the last step in an ongoing program for life. It is my duty to carry the message of hope to those who still suffer or are looking for a newer, deeper freedom. That has been, and continues to be my experience. It continues to grow. As I continue to gain faith that I will live 200 years, I am emboldened to live my dreams. Already I have lived far beyond that which was promised. The fact that I have been able to see my oldest son turn 24, and have reared four children has been a real joy. My daughter is 27 at this writing, and the other two sons are 22 and 15 at this writing. That is indeed a true miracle and I thank God for the opportunity.

I have been blessed to have seen my sister married and rearing three children. I am watching my nephew and nieces grow and have been able to start the healing process that the ancestors would have us continue. That process is manifesting in my relationship with my mother, which has evolved into one that is loving and nurturing. We have always loved each other, but our relationship has matured a great deal over time. I have also watched as she, after over 70 years, has begun to heal a wound of resentment that she has had with her father since before his death long, long ago. I have been able to do some of the healing work with her and I am sure that her healing is proving to be of great benefit to our entire family. My mother is a cancer survivor from way back. In the early part of 1990, she was diagnosed with colon cancer and underwent a resection operation where part of her colon was taken out. She then underwent chemotherapy and has been healed ever since. My sister Pam has not gone untouched by physical challenges.

Though unable to conceive children biologically with her husband Anthony, they are raising three children in spite of being afflicted by a pulmonary degenerative disease called sarcoidosis. The disease is also one that affects the immune system and it causes her to cough uncontrollably at times. In spite of it all, she possesses a determination that is characteristic of the members of our family. I guess it is in the genes.

I have visited Africa, India, Europe, Hawaii….been all over the Caribbean and the United States. I have traveled in search of health and peace of mind and have found both. I have had many wonderful years of marriage to a woman that I consider to be a queen. Dionne has stood by my side and been true to the vows that we have taken—until death do us part. I have had the simple pleasures of spending time at my children's basketball or football practices and games. I have been blessed to participate in my daughter's wedding, the children's various graduations and so much more.

I have lived my dream of being a radio announcer and D.J. and am currently living the dream of being a writer and television producer. I have jumped from an airplane from 13,000 feet and have purveyed the exquisitely beautiful coral reef of the Pacific and the Caribbean. All these things are beautiful, but there is still so much more that I would love to do. Though some might consider being afflicted with these various diseases to be tragic, it has been a catalyst for me to live my life more fully. There have been many times when fear has tried to overcome me and steal my joy. There are many life experiences that have been affected by the dynamics involved with the keen sense of mortal awareness that is a part of facing supposed death. The point is that there also is opportunity in having to live life in that way. I realized that the truth of the matter is that no one is going to get out of this thing alive!

There was a time when I had been afraid to live and scared to die! I have come to understand that the only way to heal fear is with love. Love heals all. God is love and we are best served when we surrender to God, surrender to love, surrender to heal.

***

I long to carry this message of hope to those that want it. Finally, it has been revealed to me that the way to change the world, is to begin with first changing the one. That one being I can change is myself. Then by that example, I could begin to have the prayer to be "a vessel of His word, and an instrument of Her will" be answered. And so it is. So be it.

A turning point in my life most certainly was when I was blessed to find a better way of life. When I was airlifted from the battlefield of life and resuscitated, it breathed new life into a corpse that had been left for dead on the scrap heap of humanity. I had to learn a more simple way of life if my life was to be spared. It was then that I learned the meaning of gratitude and began to incorporate it into my daily perspective of life. It would seem that I have been granted a reprieve and a Purple Heart by the real Commander in Chief—God!! As a benefit of this great honor, I have granted a daily reprieve based on the maintenance of my spiritual condition. There are things that I do to maintain that benefit. I will tell you about that in a moment.

Another turning point (besides meeting my wife and having my children), was finding out that I was HIV positive. Though I have generally maintained a positive attitude, there have been times when I have suffered grave emotional upheavals. It was at these times that I have been most compelled towards change. I can honestly say that I am glad to have had the experience of living with these diseases because they have been the most forceful impetus towards me enjoying the quality of life I am not sure I would have experienced without them.

I have been, and still am, very motivated towards enjoying life. I believe that I have a true understanding of what "a day at a time" means. I have come to know that we create our own reality. So, whatever my experience, it is what I attracted in order to fulfill my destiny, of which I am constantly free to choose. Everything begins with a thought. Writing this book is a wonderful example of that. I am also motivated to create even greater freedom for others and myself. Now I feel like I am healed enough to join in on the reconnaissance missions back into the battle zones in an attempt to help save some of the others who are fighting to be free. This time, though, I do not have to fight alone, and I have some artillery to fight with. Moreover, ultimately and paradoxically, it is the lesson of surrender that it would seem that we humans come to the planet to learn and share. It is in surrendering that we finally win.

Another turning point worthy of special mention in this long trail of synchronicity was meeting my Sister and Brother of the Spirit, Suzanne and Muhammad Zahir. Though I have learned from many and been very close to some, it is the journey that began with the videotaping of their wedding (as per her last minute request after an obscure referral by another teacher that I had met). That has really accelerated my opportunities to evolve as a spirit having this human experience. Though I have been on a perpetual path towards enlightenment, as we all are, the love and assistance that they have provided has been life changing. The work my Sister Suzanne has done on this and other plane on my behalf is nothing short of angelic. My Brother Muhammad has shown insight, courage and compassion far beyond the call of duty. Through them both, I have been exposed to knowledge that has hastened my search for the most important knowledge of all—Knowledge of self. It is that knowledge that is the precursor to the God consciousness that I seek. I truly feel that it is what we all seek, and is our purpose here on this plane. At least one of them being to make known the unknown.

I have love for many and have had wonderful relationships along the way. I plan to write again and explore different facets of life through the eyes of many. I will get the chance to speak about my relationships with other people as I talk about the different things that have served me well in this quest towards health. Knowledge has been the most important weapon given to me. Courage has been another. Often our courage can be measured in our ability to challenge fear when faced with the opportunity to succumb to it.

***

I had one other turning point in my life that has motivated me to live my truth as best as I can. It, too, is cloaked in synchronicity and mystery. While at a business forum, where I had spent a great deal of money to be exposed to a lot of investors and information, I found myself being challenged to drop the veil that we tend to live behind so as to not be seen for who we really are for fear of judgment and rejection. Being in the midst of this business forum where it seemed important to project the best image possible in order to impress any prospective investors certainly did NOT seem like it was the time or the place to talk about the truth of my sordid past, so I was very hesitant. This forum proved that it was different and much more than I anticipated because it taught co-operative business as opposed to competition. A part of the lesson was learning how to identify and crystallize one's real, true message and purpose. I was compelled to volunteer as an example. I still don't remember why. I certainly did not have to be picked. A man named Joel Roberts, who was touted as the best media coach in the land, was leading the session. His work thus far was impeccable, but I was looking for a way to engage the learning process and create a higher profile there at the seminar in order to increase my opportunities to realize my desire to create a multimedia production company. I got high profile all right.

After a minute of friendly grilling, like a producer for a TV or radio show would do, this gentleman had extracted a great deal of what I considered to be personal information. I thought divulging these things about myself in this environment would ruin my chances for any positive results, and would mean a waste of the rest of my time and money. The session was at the beginning of the forum and I was sure that being one of only a couple of black people there was going to be a liability. I ended up telling him and the audience that I was from the South Side of Jamaica Queens, that I had shot dope and that though I was dressed up and looking quite GQ, I was raised in the ghetto. I explained that the things that I had seen and lived had given me a unique perspective on life, and that I wanted to help change the way the world viewed the kind of experience. I explained that I was that one in one hundred that escaped from the grips of addiction and rose above the battlefields of life. Joel extracted that information from me and then he put it into a perspective that was graphic and moving. The whole thing was being videotaped. The thing is, by the time he was finished with story, it was eloquently vivid and evocative. There was not one dry eye in the audience of over two hundred.

It was a special moment for the both of us, as well as all who attended. It dropped my personal veil that I often hide behind for social acceptance. For many of us who where there, it gave us all a new freedom to share our truths and gave us all more courage to be honest and vulnerable. It changed the tenor of the rest of the forum, and garnered me more love and respect than I could have imagined (or believed). Many people came to me with their own personal stories, and all at once, I felt like I was in my element. I was overwhelmed with love.

It was then that I began to understand more fully the power of living one's truth. I had known before, but had never experienced something so provocative. As it was said by that gentleman Joel Roberts, whom I now call friend, "You people (with valuable life experiences) are retreating from your own greatness." I am not sure where I am going, but I have to go. I am being compelled to tell my story. I have stopped using the word try, and I work towards not categorizing things as either right or wrong. It has been my experience that right and wrong is relative to time and place. All of the variables are fluid and interchangeable. To box myself in, or limit myself by those beliefs, as can happen with the way we perceive religion, education, or anything else, is counterproductive to the attainment of freedom. I think that it is important to keep an open mind.

That is not to say that we need not use certain parameters as we gain greater discipline and knowledge of self. We probably need those parameters as banisters on the stairway of life. I am evolving into a newer state of freedom that allows me to more fully experience the adventure of life. I am less of a spectator and more of a player, not bent on the outcome of the game so much as being immersed in the enjoyment of playing. Sure, there is joy in "winning," but there, too, is as great a joy in giving an assist that will help someone else get in the game. It would seem that is how teams usually win. Separation is an illusion. We are all the same team.

So the lesson continues. At this writing, I am 47years old. In the past few years I have begun to play basketball competitively again, after a 10-year (at least) lay off. Michael Jordan doesn't have anything on me. Nor does another man that I greatly admire—Magic Johnson. He, too, has seemed to enjoy the adventure of life, and has had the courage and dignity that has inspired many, including me. I am sure that people probably believe that Magic Johnson has done so well with his journey having HIV because he has lots of money. It probably helps to be able to access the best that money can buy, but I am here to prove that it is more than just having money that will save those who are challenged by anything in life. Magic will surely tell you that it is about attitude, lifestyle, how you think and the level of participation in your own survival. My desire is to live as useful a life as possible, one day at a time. I know these things are possible, and even probable, as long as I remember who the Supreme Commander is and who it is I am fighting the war for. Actually, I no longer fight the war because I have surrendered. Someday we will all be free.

A NEW ATTITUDE

Lifestyle change is a very important aspect of changing the behaviors that contribute to disease and their proliferation. First things first. I had to learn how to say "NO THANK YOU" to the first drink or drug—and be comfortable saying it. For that there are many kinds of treatment and therapy. I have had a few, and I would suggest that anyone experiencing substance abuse of any kind seek out a Twelve Step Program. For even greater transition and healing from the emotional and mental trauma that comes from living with HIV/AIDS, I suggest the 12 step support program called HIV Anonymous. Even after having been in the 12 step recovery programs for drug addiction and alcoholism and having been clean and sober through the use of the program, I still got great benefit from practicing the 12 steps of HIVA (see the end of the book for more details). It has helped me to be more courageous about living. It has helped me to have the courage to disclose my status with my family and the world.

Disclosure is an issue that each person who is diagnosed will have to deal with one way or the other. Of course, whether a person decides to tell anyone that you are not putting at direct risk should be entirely up to you. If you are seriously considering having sexual relations and you know that you are HIV positive, it is a responsibility to have an honest conversation with that person about the risk they are taking and give them the opportunity to make an informed choice as to whether or not to do that. That is a scary proposition for most, because it means risking rejection. It means the possibility of not being able to be loved or get sex. As quiet as it is kept, most people who have had risky behavior and are at risk of being infected don't want to know if they are exposed and carrying the disease because they do not want to have to be either responsible for their behavior and risk the possibility of a lifetime of sexually responsible behavior. There is also a great deal of legally precarious situations for those who do not disclose their positive status to their partner. Personally, I think it is not fair to legislate even irresponsible sexual behavior, but I do think that we have a responsibility to our sexual partners. More importantly, people are responsible for protecting themselves, and unless a person is being raped and engaging in a sexual act without consent, it is each individual's personal responsibility to protect themselves from disease to the best of their ability. That means using protection and having the conversation with our partner before having sex. I did not share my status with very many people for many different reasons. I wanted to protect myself, my family, especially my mother, wife and children, from the hypocrisy and ignorance of society in general. Also, I am blessed to be loved by a lot of people. I believe the power of love to be formidable, to say the least. It was my belief that the fear of my death, in a powerful way, by many of the people that loved me, would create a negative effect on the universe, and their fear of my death would cause everyone more worry than was needed. People were a lot more fearful then. Now, society has an easier time dealing with this disease, especially since the medicines began prolonging life. HIV Anonymous will also help many people transition through the difficult choices we have to make when we are HIV positive. Either way, I am more willing now to talk about my experience because of my personal transition and I have experienced both pain and great freedom.

WHEN THE LEVEL OF HONESTY RISES, THE DEPTH OF THE RELATIONSHIP INTENSIFIES.

MEDICAL MUST

It is extremely important to find a good doctor who has knowledge and experience in treating HIV. It was my first Doctor that whipped my ass into fighting shape. I heard about Dr. Barbara Justice listening to my favorite radio announcer, Imhotep Gary Byrd, on WLIB in New York. I always got great information listening to his radio show, and he has been a role model for the type of radio personality I aspired to be. Dr. Justice was talking about the different things she was doing in the field of AIDS research and it sounded radical and hopeful, so I went to her office to check it out. Dr. Barbara was a powerful influence and a great doctor, as well as a fine spirit. She was a good-looking sister as well, and that did not hurt at all. The first thing she had me do was quit smoking, something I had been doing since I was 14 years old. I had considered stopping my smoking but was having a hard time doing so.

I remember having the courage and asking my father for permission to smoke, and he told me no. His reasoning was that if I started smoking I would soon be smoking pot and then be using hard drugs. I thought that was insane reasoning then, but when I chose to smoke in spite of his wise advice, it ironically turned out that he was right, flat out right. I ended up living his vision. Unfortunately, quitting smoking was harder to quit than heroin. I was much more physically and mentally addicted to cigarettes than anything else.

I had to wean myself off cigarettes, and it took about a year of back and forth before I was finally shamed into surrender by Dr. Barbara. I had to ask God to remove the compulsion and obsession to smoke cigarettes, just as She had taken the desire for heroin and cocaine from me. Dr. Justice is a strong Black woman, with great energy and will. She had many famous patients and the promise of access to cutting edge treatments. These treatments were not readily available, especially in the Black community, better known as the front lines. Moreover, Dr. Justice represented a greater level of hope in my mind. She threatened that if I did not stop smoking she would no longer treat me—plain and simple. I quit smoking not long after. I want to live, and at the time, Dr. Justice was my best hope. She turned out to be a good friend as well as a great Doctor.

MEDICAL SUGGESTIONS

Find a doctor that you can feel comfortable with and that you believe has experience and information with THIS disease. I have since oved to another state and have another doctor, Dr. William Richardson, whom I have become comfortable with. I have done some of my own research, but then I usually take it to him to see if I am on the path that will serve me best.

***

Find a doctor that will be a coach for you and encourage you to do the things that are in your interest. At first I was leery of my new doctor, but it was because I was slow to trust a new doctor, and I was still living privately with this disease, so the way his staff dealt with my privacy was important. After all, I had moved, in part, to start over new. I did not want the "stigma" of being positive to hinder my growth, or become an excuse for my inability to grow.

***

Create a partnership with your doctor. Do the research that will allow you to make informed decisions with your health care professional. The Internet is filled with enough knowledge about this and any other issue. I have sometimes had to have the courage to overrule my doctor's advice and thus far it has worked out well for me. I have been able to do it comfortably by having the information and following my own intuition. It is a scary thing to do, especially when your doctor and most conventional wisdom point to doing one thing and your intuition and desire is to do something different. Each person is different and we are ultimately responsible for our own choices.

***

Just like it took a while for me to figure out that I was my parents' first child and that they did not know it all, the same is true for us as "infected" people. The medical profession is still learning about this disease and we can help them by being conscious, honest, informed and wise.

SEXUAL RELATIONS

H ere is where there can be real trouble. There was a feeling of being tainted, less than, out of God's favor, not lovable, and more. There was a fear that no one would ever want to have sex with a person that could give her a virus that could kill them! If my sexual partner is HIV negative—then what does the HIV positive do? Does either partner decide to stay or go?? If not, will the positive person have to tell everyone else that they want to have intimate relations with that I am HIV positive or that I have AIDS, hence risking rejection and public scrutiny?? What if the positive person has not yet disclosed to family and friends and is not in a committed relationship? How does one handle having sex with a person you may not trust with such sensitive information for fear that if things ever got bad in the relationship that person might try to use the personal information as some kind of leverage? Am I going to have to be abstinent for the rest of my life, or am I going to have to find someone else who is also positive and pursue a relationship with her? There are many questions about sex that I wanted to answer. I had no idea how it would turn out. I imagined that if I were going to be single, and have to tell someone else about my "secret," I would do so in a way that would allow the person to be forewarned. I would make them aware that they were dealing with a person that was in the highest of risks, and most probably exposed. That way I could maintain my privacy;

yet feel morally absolved and responsible for my actions. There is nothing like the freedom of being open and honest about our status and what our true sexual behavior is. The truth will set you free. Counseling can be an important help in finding the strength to deal with these and the many other questions and situation that arise from being HIV positive. There are a great deal of support groups and organizations where people can get information about how people are dealing with these issues. It is very helpful to not have to deal with being positive alone. It is also ludicrous for anyone to engage in risky sexual behavior without taking responsibility for his or her own well-being. That does not absolve the person that is "positive" from giving his partner the option of choosing not to have sex. We should all assume that this virus is living in all of us. That way, we are all responsible for how we protect ourselves. It would come down to that anyway. After all is said and done, it does not matter who or how this virus is contracted. Only the fact that it does exist in our universe holds meaning.

***

For me, the question was more about being deserving of love and sex. I could not understand why my wife would stick around with all that was at risk for her. I did not feel deserving of that kind of love, and quite honestly was somewhat suspect at the motives behind it. That was years ago. I have learned to feel more worthy, but it is a work in progress. It has always been a serious concern about me infecting my wife. I know that we are responsible and have use a condom 98% of the time we have been aware of my status. She has been tested since the last time we were irresponsible and has still maintained her negative status. We have been able to practice perfect adherence since then. The last thing I would want is to infect anyone else, especially her. We have been extremely blessed and I thank God for the courage and love that my wife has shown.

Sexual conduct is the behavior that we want to control if we are going to slow or stop the proliferation of this and other sexually transmitted diseases. Sexual behavior is why how have created this epidemic. It is a manifestation of our desire to be free from uncontrolled attitudes and behaviors, not the least of which is our unchecked sexual appetites.

There is no room for judgment in these matters. It is important to strive towards responsibility on a daily basis. If one should fall short of the glory of God, it is more productive to keep a positive outlook, than it is to dwell in guilt and shame. These are the things that disease feeds off of, and fear and judgment are counterproductive to a healing state of mind. We sometimes want to beat ourselves up to satisfy a secret desire to feel guilty. I have always said, "I would rather be faking than really be sick." I have also said, "It is one thing to play the role, but don't let the role play you!" We should definitely strive to act in a way that takes responsibility for our sexual behavior. We should also know that we create our realities on more than one level, and that our attitude about any action is as important as the act itself. The effect that it has on our state of mind, affects each and every cell in our bodies.

***

I know from personal experience that we can think or "guilt" ourselves into bad health. There was a period of time when I had been living like there was no tomorrow. The next thing I looked up and it was 10 years since I had been diagnosed and not only had I survived, but I had not even been sick. A lot of my friends had died from the disease.

I had enjoyed my life and was not really concerned with anything except my growing personal freedom. I had achieved some level of personal freedom partly because I had no real worry about things like my credit and saving money. Then, 10 years later, I was not that martyr that subconsciously I thought I would be. I mean, even though I told myself that I wanted to live, I subconsciously knew that it was more likely that I would not. Though my relationship with my loved ones and others was built on my desire for creating independence for them and freedom for me, I needed to shift into something else, or I would manifest the death and doom that I had secretly coveted as an excuse for living recklessly. Death is the easier way out, and a great reason to not be concerned about long-term financial situations. Impending death has a way of making living in the present more attractive than usual.

In a way, it was just like when I was using drugs. When I was shooting dope and coke, I would always justify stealing or spending all my money on satisfying my desire to be free. The fact was that I expected to "kill myself" each time I used or got to the end of a vicious drug run and was broke and guilty, so it did not matter what I did to get the drugs. My intention was to not be alive to face the consequences anyway. Obviously, the fact that I would always survive that self-deception and insanity was a source of real frustration. I am glad now that I survived, but that kind of guilt made me wish that I were dead.

Now, in a sense, even though I was clean and sober, I was looking for the easy way out again. Death this time would give me the way out, but I would be absolved of the responsibility of actually creating my own death. That would be the pass I would need when going through the life review with God. He would know that it was out of my hands. There was just one thing. In this chess game with God, I was totally unprepared for the moves She would put on me, again. As like before, with the drugs and all, this part of life would serve to be a great lesson and a blessing. Life would not be that easy to forfeit for me.

The fact is, though, that while thinking in this way, I was telling my body, my cells and my mind that I wanted to be sick and die. That would be the only way to fulfill the scenario that I had certainly envisioned. There was quite a battle going on inside, when I look back at it. The dichotomy was that I knew that I would need a positive outlook to be healed. I wanted to be well, and stick around to see what was going to happen in life with the maturing of my children, my growth with my wife, and to see how close I could come to God while here in the body.

It was then that I realized two things. One was the power of the mind, and the other was the fact that everything happens for a reason. I had been thinking my way into bad health in order to fulfill my unconscious prophecy, and before I knew it, I had wished myself into being diagnosed as having full blown AIDS. My T-cell count, the cells that are measured as a supposed indicator of our body's ability to fight of infection, was down to 4. Anything lower than 200 is considered to indicate full-blown AIDS. I began to start manifesting other indications of the disease such as thrush, wasting and other types of infections. It was then that the God consciousness intensified and my spirit's will to live kicked in. I know that that spirit that activates this body for the purpose of having this human experience was not done yet with the experience.

Not only that, but the freedom that I desired as a basic necessity, was to be further enhanced by this experience. It was because I was diagnosed as being full blown, that I was able to retire from my job and get my pension. That pension, is, at the very least, enough to take care of my real needs. My real needs are a roof over the heads of myself and my family, and food in our tummies. That happened because I desired to create freedom with such intensity that it had to manifest. The crazy part is that I would think myself into bad health in order for that same freedom to happen.

So, this is the paradox of life. We create our reality, but we do so on at least a few levels of consciousness. There was/is my conscious desire for personal freedom and my unconscious desire for that freedom to come from death, which my mind saw as the ultimate freedom. I believe that nothing happens by mistake, and that the situations we create occur in order for us learn the lesson needed to evolve as a spirit. The evolution is but one step in the process of the re-galvanization of all souls. Redefined, our separateness is but an illusion. We are all a part of the evolution of spirit.

So, it would seem that this was an opportunity for me to learn some great lessons. Situations and circumstances that are of our creation anyway, are an opportunity to evolve. We do so by practicing knowledge gained from prior experiences—and when truly wise—from the experience of others.

One of the lessons I learned from this experience was the power of thought. It is no coincidence that after getting some relief from this knowledge, the universe would open up more opportunities for greater knowledge about these things. I realized that not only was I playing the role, but the role was playing me....right out of the pocket!! I was truly deserving of being retired due to my status—but I did not want to die to prove it.

I believe that our thoughts are the precursor to any creation and are the tool of God, who resides within each and every one of us at the lower cerebellum. With my thoughts I had finally orchestrated a reality that had created a measure of freedom. Now, I needed to separate myself from the role by giving greater clarity to what I was creating. I needed to be able to regain a positive state of mind by accepting life and enjoying the experience. This psychic change was necessary in order to begin again, the healing process. That process would be to relate a positive "state of mind." That attitude would be translated to the cells in my body, which in and of themselves act as millions of tiny little minds. It also affected the way I would be able to transmit and receive information from and to the universe. That is what makes a holistic approach so important. The process of changing my thoughts became the most important "way of being" in the "recovery" process.

This time it was the evolution of the knowledge that I had gained from the experience getting clean and sober. It was my experience from that other life changing reality that I had created in an effort to attain that recurring desire—the will to be free. I had the opportunity to evolve by applying that knowledge to this experience. At the core of my desire to grow is the will to live. That will, I believe, is God's gift to man. I practiced using the "Serenity Prayer" as an affirmation. It goes:

> God, grant me the serenity to accept the things I cannot change, the courage to change the things I can, and the wisdom to know the difference.

That prayer continued to remind me of my powerlessness to change what had already been. As my level of acceptance grew, so did my level of serenity. It gave me the courage to believe that I could and would be healed. As I became more courageous, I was more inclined to believe that I would live 200 years. In that case, I would need to take care of this body and allow myself the luxury of actually making longer-range plans.

As time went on, I started to see the benefits of thinking positively. Not only did my health get better; my blood tests were indicating improvement, as well. I had started on the new triple cocktail therapy around that time. I resisted taking any medication, depending rather on more natural remedies. It took me creating this dire of a reality before I found it necessary to "resign" myself to taking what I thought to be not only toxic medications, but also creating a prison that I would have to live in. I saw it as taking away my freedom and challenging my self-discipline. I did not know if the medications would work. If they did, I did not want to be a slave to them. It turns out that it is all about attitude. While I was taking the miracle cocktails that my doctor suggested, my blood showed no discernable trace of the virus. As long as I took the medicine the way it was prescribed, it seemed to work in the way it was supposed to work.

I changed my attitude to believe that the medications would help me to heal because I was in perfect position to be healed. I had to believe that the reason why I thrive is because I had proven that I had the will to live. By not going back to drugs when God removed the obsession and the compulsion and by quitting smoking when challenged by life to do so, and following a Path that demanded great discipline, and by "working hard to live a stress-free life," I had the best chance to be totally healed. I had survived long enough to see the creation of these "miracle drugs." My best chance now was to apply what I had learned and had been blessed to experience.

I did that to the best of my ability and it has worked,

fabulously. I take no credit for life; the gift it has been from God. Given the opportunity to live, it is our duty to do the best that we can with life. That is another lesson I have learned. By applying all of these things, I now enjoy radiant health, just for today. The subconscious desire to die still lingers, but I now understand that it is dying while living that I seek. It is what I have always been seeking. I was seeking it as a child when I drank the ink from the pen in junior high school under the pretense that I just wanted the sympathy. My desire then was bred from the frustration of not being able to change or deal with the world as it was. Simply put, I wanted to be and feel love in its purest form, as we all do. We all just want to be loved.

I was seeking God as a drug user and alcohol abuser. The quest then was the same. I wanted to still the mind and to know God. It is no coincidence that I would try to get higher and "higher." Physiologically, it can be explained that the chemical activity of the mind when using drugs has the effect of changing our consciousness—in some cases to a subconsciousness, and other's to a super consciousness. That certainly had the effect of fooling me to believe that I was on the path towards God, Death or both.

Sex had proved to be at least as seductive and alluring a possibility. I pursued the warm feeling of "love" and passion as an earthly substitute for a "heavenly" experience. My obsession and compulsion for orgasms, and the validation that comes with the acquiescence of another human being's permission to be "all up in" their body, ran neck and neck with my desire to get high. In fact, they went hand in hand. Ultimately, they were a part of the same desire, a quest to see God and lose my mind.

PERSONAL INSIGHTS

I stopped wearing a watch many years ago when I was diagnosed with HIV/AIDS. It no longer made sense for me to be preoccupied with time. Now, I enjoy watching the adventure of life unfold. I practice remembering to love in a detached manner, meaning that I am practicing giving unconditional love without being attached to the outcome. It is important for me to remember that I am responsible for the effort, and not the outcome. Not only that, but judgment of the outcome could sometimes limit my ability to evolve and grow from the experience and the wisdom that could be its culmination.

I have learned that right and wrong is relative to time and space, and that both are products of this physical plane. What may seem "wrong" at any given time, like now or in the past, could be considered "right" at a different time and could have its place in the grand scheme of things. Of course, it seemed wrong for me to abuse drugs and alcohol. My having this other disease is a direct result from that act, and would also, on the surface, seem to be a "wrong" thing to happen in my life. There are so many other variables that now would have me look at these experiences in a totally different light. Those experiences are now clearly the right thing for me to have had to experience. We have to be aware of the parameters that these judgments put around our living, but it would seem that being non-judgmental about the experience would give us a more even perspective.

Because of these "wrong" things I have experienced, I have been driven to live more closely to my innermost dreams and desires. These things may not have been attainable in any other way. All of the people, places and things that I have been exposed to would have changed had any of the things that I had experienced been different. I am astounded and amazed when I think of the synchronicity of my life, up to and including the people that called as I was writing this book. The conversations that I had with people that I had been thinking strongly about when they called mirrored the topic that I "happened" to be writing about at that moment. It was further validation that I was on the right track. It was also fun to watch a phenomenon develop that evidenced what I was learning about the connection between all things.

People, places and things played an important part in creating the situations that would induce the pain that would be the motivation for my greatest learning. The greater awareness of these things, and the role that they played in the drama, made it possible for me to short circuit the feedback loop that was dominating and directing my life until that point. It was when I changed the people, places and things in my life that I was able to begin having different experiences. These new experiences served me in a way that would allow me to move on a path on which I felt like I was growing. At least, it broke the "Twighlight Zone" repetition of the elementary lessons of life. We are here in this life to learn these lessons, and opportunities to learn them will continue to present themselves until we show the universe that we have learned the lesson. If we don't get it at first, those lessons will persist and intensify until we do.

As a seeker of knowledge and spirituality, I began to meet other people, like myself, that were in search of God, and had experienced the" hell" of not "getting it," not learning the lessons that life was trying to teach. Many of us had to be motivated by the pain of experiences like drug addiction and alcoholism before we surrendered. These new friends and associates had found a new way of living, and were very willing to share that way of life with me and anyone else that wanted it. Paradoxically, the maintenance of their sober condition and spiritual growth that made sobriety possible was contingent on their willingness to share what had been so freely given to them. They, and now I, have to "Pay It Forward."

7 WAYS TO RISE ABOVE THE BATTLEFIELDS OF LIFE

The journey of life is the opportunity to remember that we are one with the Father and with each other. Relationship is the illusion that we are separate from God, and therefore, somehow separate from each other. We are all connected, if by nothing else, by the air that we breathe. Furthermore, our ego creates a life drama surrounding this belief. Indeed, it is only a belief and not the truth, for the truth is that we are eternal and inseparable from the Creator.

As pointed out in *A Course In Miracles*, no right mind can believe that its will is stronger than God's. That, though, is the pretense that many or all conflict is built on. Be it personal conflict or the social conflict that seems to motivate the world condition we have created, it is founded on the premise that our ego is separate and in control of creation. The mind is profoundly split and afraid of the truth. This sets us up for the ongoing "search" for God and the desire to "know" what God's will for us is. It is like the dog chasing its tail. The Father and I are one. I am not the Father, but we are all made in His image.

I wrote this book to try to find a way to communicate what life has illuminated for me and allowed me to remember. My hope is that through the eyes of my experiences, you might find a spark of the light that guides us back home with God. We all must return to the Father at some point. The mystery is when will we go. After all, none of us are going to get out of this thing alive!

Fearing death can be real even if it is a bit irrational. It is a certain aspect of life. The key is to learn how to practice dying while living, and that is done by meditation. Whatever we can do to create an atmosphere for meditation is a step in the "right" direction. Pain and suffering can be the greatest teachers in our lives. That cycle of pain and suffering as teaching tools will continue until we decide to create something else as a means of ascension. The ego, which has a vested interest in perpetuating drama, illness, and other illusion, works hard to keep us from remembering that which we are. Our Will is the Will of God, and that Will is not the ego. That is why the ego is against us.

What seems to be fear of God is actually our fearful interpretation of a false reality created by the ego, much like the proverbial boogieman. Wrong perception is the wish that things be as they are not. Healing is a release from fear and an awakening to what we truly are—love. All healing involves replacing fear with love. In order to be conscious of the ego and the many ways it keeps us entangled in this game and illusion, we must internally practice surrendering to God's Will, which is the truth and the Way.

Surrender in this way is not the giving up, or making ourselves vulnerable, though our ego tells us it is. Ego will say that to keep us from removing our self from conflict. The ego enjoys the confusion, and it thrives on the drama. Left unchecked, the ego will constantly divert our attention away from the kingdom of heaven within. Realization that there is great power in surrendering, and not getting entwined in egoic warfare, is something that we all feel and realize as truth at our core level. Resistance to surrender is at the core of all conflict, and is the cause for all of what we perceive as "sickness." When we surrender to what is and operate in the now, we become present and engage the flow of what is real. The past is not real, nor is the future. Only now is real. Our level of serenity is directly proportionate to our level of acceptance of what is.

I have had to remember (learn) that I am responsible for the way thoughts are made manifest in my life. My health is a manifestation of the thoughts that I have had. It had been a reflection of the control that my ego has had on my way of being. I have since (learned) remembered that good health begins with the relinquishing of all attempts to use the body lovelessly, and the beginning of the proper perspective on life under God's guidance. I merely need remember that regularly in order to maintain the attitude that will serve as the foundation for good mental, emotional and physical health.

There are some affirmations I use to remind myself to remember who I am, so I can remain conscious of who I am being. I learned them while attending the School for Enlightenment, a place where many experience the teachings of Ramtha, a 35,000-year-old male spirit channeling through the body of a middle aged white woman. The core of the teachings is to help us remember the true divinity we, as children of God, truly can be. And so it is. So be it.

I create this day from the Lord God of my being.
I am lawgiver and whatsoever I speaketh manifest straightaway.

1. I am filled with the power of my spirit. I acknowledge a Higher Power and seek ways to remain conscious of that power. "I laugh and I joke, but I do not play" I like to say.

By surrendering to a loving, merciful and omnipotent God of my understanding, I am empowered.

Stress kills and I work hard at living a stress free life. It is very important to be positive about life and to find the good in it. It is good to be pragmatic and acknowledge the world for what it is, but we should not loose our attitude of optimism and acceptance. It serves us well to expect miracles to happen in our lives and the lives of others. Complimenting others is also a part of the power of our spirit. When finding the good in others and sharing that good with them and others is done sincerely, it is healing.

2. I am filled with joy. Practice surrender to the God of our understanding. Gratitude, acceptance and tolerance are characteristics to be practiced. Joy is a by-product of practicing universal laws. Smiling and laughter help enhance our joy on this plane. My joy is multiplied when I share it with others.

3. I am aware of my past. We should learn from our life experiences. Even greater wisdom can come from learning from the experiences of others. There are many ways to gain knowledge. What we focus on with our minds soon becomes a part of our thinking. Reading enlightening material is empowering and has its way of creating opportunity for us to enrich our minds. That knowledge affects how we experience our world.

It also gives us clues as to how we can ascend, or rise above the battlefields of life. Knowledge is power, but knowledge applied is wisdom.

Conflict and struggle has always distracted us from the greater good. Surrender and tolerance help us to avoid being caught in the whirlpool of confusion, leaving more time for us to create an atmosphere of prayer, meditation and love.

4. I call forth new adventures to experience this day. Yesterday is history and tomorrow is still a mystery; our joy is manifest in the clarity of our focus on today. "We must become like little children" it is said in the bible. I enjoy experiencing the adventure of life. I enjoy watching the adventure unfold like a wonderful movie that we are both participants and observers. I practice being detached from the outcome of life's situations, while engaging life in a loving manner. Progress, not perfection in this area is the goal. Remembering that I am always responsible for the effort and not the outcome, relieves me of the belief that I am in charge of the universe. That is God's job and I am glad. There are consequences to my behavior, and certain immutable universal laws that it would behoove me to adhere to. The law of karma dictates that in this world of polarity which is identified and good and bad, positive and negative, as well as right and wrong; every action has an equal and opposite reaction. Our motives should always be colored by love.

5. I am healed this day. We are what we eat. If we are to invite the greatest guest, God, into our conscious living, should not we clean up a little? We should prepare a place for Her in the way that your heart makes apparent. Habits that are not conducive to optimum health detract from our life experience and make us slaves to our own desires. Those desires are often created from tradition, or by those who would benefit from our perpetuation of those habits. They do not serve us or the universe and we should work towards applying the discipline needed to change our behavior.

6. All things I create this day, I accept their manifestation and their experience. There is a loving God that has created all things and the wonder of this creation is amazing. We are said to be made in the image of God, hence we , too, have the capacity to create. That is evident in our ability to procreate our species. We also create through thoughts. Everything begins with a thought, then it is manifest through our efforts. Emotions affect our ability to actualize our thoughts in different ways. Being able to experience our emotions, yet apply a set of principles towards our actions helps to create the discipline needed to practice Christ-like behavior. Jesus was the example of this. He came so that we may know that it is possible for us to achieve this even while in the flesh. There are no coincidences in this world and everything has purpose.

7.   I am and give abundant love.

These affirmations help me to maintain proper communication with the Holy Spirit, which is the Voice for Life Itself. As Earth, Wind and Fire said in the song "That's The Way of the World," A child is born with a heart of gold, way of the world makes his heart so cold." At that moment of creation, we are endowed with a spark of life, a spark of divinity. From that subatomic particle which was manifest as thought in our parents and the Original Thought in the Mind of God, we have evolved. We are forever linked with all things in and out of Creation by the commonality of the elements of our creation. We are joined eternally by their origin, to which we all ultimately return, as does the rain to the sea.

I acknowledge the soul to be the recorder of life. It traverses the illusion of time and space, and shapes the way we are to create choices. We choose between what we know to be, and what the ego tells us we should want it to be. The body exists in a world of mind with two voices fighting for its possession. In this way, the body is seen as being capable of making the concepts of both health and sickness meaningful. In reality, we know that we are like God and not limited to the body. Therefore, we can transcend the illusion of sickness by going beyond the limitations of the body and remembering with the Will of God—our truth.

There is a revelation that I (learned) remembered when my father was killed. I had the chore of going to the morgue to identify his body. While looking at the corpse that he had left behind, I realized that the life that was my father was no more in the flesh. The corpse was just the mortal coil that he had co-created and used to work on this plane. The life force, that spark of life was now withdrawn, and the flesh consigned to returning to the elements from which it came. Ashes to ashes, dust to dust. That was a defining moment for me. It was then that I was able to begin to look beyond the illusion that the ego creates to keep us distracted and doing. It was then I began to realize that life is about being—humans being, not humans doing, as we are fooled into believing.

It was then that I came to remember that God's Will for me is complete peace and joy. I had always been seeking to be in this perfect state of being through external things like the pleasures and escape of sex and drugs. These only worked momentarily, yet the promise of those moments were enough to motivate me to become a slave of my desires, therefore a slave of the ego. It could be said that ego is an acronym for "easing God out". It could also be analogized that the ego is the Satan we read about and understand as the negative force in our universe. That would conceptualize the battle between good and evil on a level of the microcosm, as the difference between God and Satan is explained on the level of the macrocosm. It would also give clues to why we often choose to do and be things that do not serve our true purpose. It would begin to explain how we, through the power of choice, often chosen sin over love. The awareness of this battle for our souls and minds makes extrication from the battlefield possible. Awareness is the first step. Faith in an unseen God, and a child-like heart, help us to circumvent the traps of the intellect and the ego. It is then we can surrender to heal.

As a part of the need to find a way of creating freedom, there are levels of thought that desire a way out of the rat race of life on this plane. On all levels of thought and being, I acknowledged that desire. Though we all have the desire to leave this plane of existence and return to our true home at the feet of the Father, we often do not acknowledge it because the thought is quickly associated with death. That is another trick of the ego. God and our life force are completely out of our control. No one has lived forever in the same body, so it is inevitable that we must leave this world eventually. God knows when that will be. Fear of death is another very powerful tool of the Devil or lower power. It may be satans' most powerful tool.

The blessing is that a paradox of life is that we can, as Jesus did, die while living. That is what was being alluded to in the explanation of the resurrection. It is what Jesus was explaining to His disciples, and what he proved by his death and rebirth. He explained that "greater works than these..." are we capable. Many people have had near death experiences and come back to this plane of life to share the experience. That does not make them Jesus, but they certainly feel blessed to return. We can learn much from the apparent uniformity of their accounts of those "near" death experiences.

I now know that it was that thought that is responsible for the manifestation of HIV/AIDS showing up in my life. I accept the responsibility for its creation to the extent that we all create our own reality. My choices have been based on my limited knowledge and perceptions. I don't blame myself for my situation, but by accepting my role in the universal scheme of things, I am healed. I do not take credit for the healing, nor do I take the blame for the situation. I simply surrender to what is. There have been choices that I have had to make about my life and my attitude that have been shaped by this part of my adventure. This has been the "cross" that I have had to bear, but that is why the situations that are our lives are created. It is so we can learn from them. Resistance is futile, for what is—is. Whatever will be—already is. My choice is to make life's situations something from which I will build on and grow from.

Moreover, I choose to not be attached emotionally to HIV/AIDS, alcoholism or drug addiction as a manifestation. I choose to grow beyond the diagnosis, and to identify with the state of Grace that is natural for a Son of God. That does not imply a state of denial about my situation. It does not mean that there are not moments when fear attempts to capture me and make me more vulnerable to it. Quite to the contrary, being conscious of the lessons that fear gives us the opportunity to learn and acting accordingly by applying love; which is the only true antidote, is not only prudent, but is necessary as an ingredient for healing. Being conscious of that Grace, and staying present by surrendering to what is, we are able to identify when the ego attempts to get us caught up in its web of deceit. Whenever I am being judgmental, needing to prove that you are wrong or that I am right, comparing myself to others or my perception of the things we have, I am being unconscious and operating in the will of ego. I no longer need to experience the pain and suffering that we humans usually create by being slaves to our desires. For that reason, I practice creating an atmosphere for the kind of healing that is ours to be. We need only remember.

So, surrendering is not giving up anything or becoming submissive to the world. We still have to live in the world. We can live in the world but not be of it. It is not the outer world that I am speaking of when I say that we are to surrender to heal. We still exist in the physical realm, and have to interact with other humans who may or may not be conscious of their actions or their own existence. We are not to be doormats. When we are able to remember to face fear and confusion with love, we change ourselves, those souls we interact with, and thereby we are changing the universe and shifting the paradigm. It is the inner world, that place where the mind is too powerful for us to exclude it, that we are to operate. We must go beyond mind, emotion and the illusion of separation in order to evolve. We can never exclude ourselves from our thoughts, at least until, through meditation, we still the mind. The more we try to fight with our thinking, or use denial as a defense, the more entangled we become in the ego's web. Letting go and letting God is the only answer.

There is a principle that we use in 12-step programs that is a reflection of a universal law and a great spiritual truth. We say, "You can't keep it unless you give it away." The paradox of life is that you must give away, freely and unconditionally, the love and knowledge that you would and have already received if it is to be replenished. Love is always there, but there is no way to have it except by giving it. This is the law of God, and it has no exceptions. What we do not give to our brother, we ourselves shall lack—not because it is not there, but because we are not aware of it as a result of our denying it in another. We are, in that case, acknowledging lack and limitation. Doing so hinders our ability to access the abundance of the universe. The principle is tied to our material situations and our relationship with money. It is a great lesson to learn because wealth can help, or hinder, our desire and ability to create an atmosphere of healing.

SEEKING SPIRITUALITY

The most important part of healing is connecting with a higher power. That is the one thing that I would consider to be an indispensable aspect of healing. Here in the West, people are becoming more aware of the power of the mind. It is the body's natural ability to heal itself. Prayer and meditation help create the atmosphere for the mind to tap into that power that is greater than us. We do, however, have to participate in our own survival.

I always believed in God. I just did not have the proper context with which to compare and verify my relationship with Her. When I was very young, I knew I was to honor my mother and father, but I felt guilty because I did not like some of the things that they did. I loved them both, though, and was hurt by the fact that they sometimes did not think that I truly loved them. They used to say that as a way of trying to get me to act in a particular way. I would have felt guilty if I did not love them. So, my love for them, as it was for the God of my understanding then, was born from fear of not being moral or Christ-like. As I matured, or grew up, and went through all my experiences, I remained "God fearing." I resisted any organized religion because I did not want to get caught up in any dogma or rituals. I also did not trust the interpretation of the Bible to anyone else. I knew that I was too lazy to read the Bible myself, and was not that sure that reading the Bible would satisfy my seeking. I still have not read the Bible, but I no longer "fear" God either. My relationship with God is one of love, admiration and respect. I have joined a wonderful church, Turner Chapel, AME located in Marietta, Georgia. I love and appreciate the power and the pleasure of worshiping there, and the opportunities to serve God and my community. I respect and admire the efforts of our congregation to be a part of the healing of the community and the world; doing so under the guidance and tutelage of Pastors Kenneth and Casandra Marcus. I really love the spirit and sound of the choir, of which my wife and mother in law are members.

I have been initiated on a Path that is centered in Eastern Philosophy for the past 15 years. Before that I was in a 12-step program that showed me how to develop a relationship with a Higher Power. As I developed that relationship, I felt compelled to be baptized. Then, after finding (or being led to) the Path, I practiced meditation as a way of knowing God and finding peace.

I am sure that meditation has had an effect on the healing process. I am sure that this healing has taken place on planes that are beyond this one, where the vibratory rate is faster than this physical plane. It seems that in meditation we are able to tap into the planes that vibrate more quickly, and from there we can create our reality through focused intent. It is from there that we can make known the unknown.

Spirituality, for me, has been found in the wonderment of God's creation and the beauty of nature. There is a level of gratitude that has been enhanced by the knowledge of my health situation. It helped me to acknowledge the fragility of life and its tenuous nature has been accentuated by the many deaths of others in similar situations I have survived.

I have had the pleasure of connecting with the beauty of nature in many places. It is everywhere, of course. Some places are more beautiful than others, to me. I am glad to have moved from New York to Georgia. There is much more green and space here. It is changing, though. I have really enjoyed spending time in the Caribbean, especially Jamaica, and Hawaii. I have visited them both whenever I could.

Actually, a great deal of the traveling I have done has been because I did not see the reason to wait to go. That time might not ever come. Conversely, It is through traveling and spending time in these island paradises that has helped to heal my spirit. Being free is the key for me. It is becoming more evident that stress is a factor in the quality of life. My level of serenity has a direct correlation to my ability to be well. "I work hard at living a stress free life."

I travel whenever I can, to places where I can relax and enjoy nature. That is one of the ways that I create an atmosphere for healing. The pictures of these beautiful places are the pictures that I call on to feed my cells and my spirit healthy pictures. Even if I can't afford to get away, I will find a way to get with nature. That is a way for me to enhance my spirituality and feel connected with the Creator.

LIVING A PROGRAM

I cannot begin to express the value of having a program to live by. Before the 12-step program, I was living in an abstract manner. Since then, I have had something to fall back on for the most basic explanations and guidance. For anyone wanting to be an active part of their own healing, getting and staying clean and sober would seem to be instrumental. I do not now, nor have I ever represented any 12 step program (except HIV Anonymous), or any other program, philosophy, religion, etc. I can only speak for myself and tell you what has worked for me thus far. That program has been the foundation for all that is serving me in my life. It is from that simple program that I have been blessed with knowledge and conscious experiences. It has given me the tools better know myself, develop a relationship with God, and peacefully co-exist with those around me. I have learned how to practice being honest, open-minded and willing to try the things that had been proven to be effective in the development of human nature. There is great benefit in working to have harmony in one's life. That is not to say that life has not put me in some situations that I would not have consciously created. Life happens. I have learned, however, that it is not what happens to you, but how you deal with what happens to you. My level of serenity is directly proportionate to my level of acceptance. It is not something that can be perfectly attained, but I am not seeking perfection, only progress. I would strongly suggest to anyone who either has a problem with drugs, alcohol, or any other addiction, to investigate the 12-step program of your choice. It would be just as advantageous for people who have no apparent substance problem, but only want to find a way to change a particular behavior or to change and improve the quality of their life. Disease is the physical manifestation of our ill thinking and subsequent behaviors and attitudes. In order to heal, we need a positive program to live by. We can create a regimen for ourselves that include all of these things as a holistic approach to creating wellness.

CHANGING DIET

When I was growing up, we ate everything. I had no problem with most of the parts of a pig. There were parts that I did not like, like the ears and toes—and the tail seemed nasty too! I would eat ham or bacon, and I even liked the smell of chitlin's. We ate just about everything. I ate ox tails, scrambled eggs and lots of other things that tasted good then. Somehow, inherently, I knew it was not good for me. I had no real vision of being disciplined in anything that I was doing, so food would not be the thing that I developed any discipline around. I believe that we create our own reality, so there must have been a part of me that wanted to be more disciplined about everything.

As a matter of fact, I remember being somewhat envious of the Five Per centers and other Muslims, Jehovah's Witness', Seventh Day Adventist and Jewish people. I would look at the way they seemed to be able to refrain from eating certain things, to live within some type of structure. I did not think that I would ever get from where I was to anywhere near where they were. That has changed with God's grace, time, and the motivation to make the best of both.

The first thing to go from my diet was alcohol and drugs. That made all the rest possible. A few years later, after accepting the Path of Sound and Light as a way of living, I stopped eating all meat, eggs, and anything made with either. I did not know at the time what God was preparing me for, but

I was intrigued with the idea of being able to see God while still in the human body. This was a part of the experiment, the one big experiment that is life. I am still experimenting with that concept, but I am sure that had I been eating meat all of these years, I may not have had as good a quality of life as I have been blessed to enjoy. Being vegetarian made me feel like I had the best chance of healing. It gave me the feeling of being disciplined. That was a feeling I had longed for secretly. Now I have gotten to live it one day at a time.

As importantly, finding a diet that serves you and doing it because you love yourself and your family, goes a long way towards the healing process. You don't have to be vegetarian, even though it has worked for me. I truly believe that the drugs that are used to keep and grow meat are contributors to the deterioration of the body. There is evidence that meat is not fully digested for long periods of time in the human body, and it actually sits in the colon and gets putrefied. Those poison toxins slowly help to destroy various organs and systems in the body. I suggest regular colon cleanses and/or enemas as a way of cleansing the colon. Colonic irrigations are something I have used occasionally as a way of cleansing my colon. When changing one's nutritional habits it is very important to get rid of the years of garbage that is laying there in the colon. It is estimated that there can be five to fifteen pounds of waste in the colon and that is what causes some to be overweight and toxic. Toxicity affects everything that we are including the way that we think.

There are many diseases that seem to be proliferating in these times. It is not hard to trace the contributing factors to diet and lack of exercise. Our immune system is enhanced by regular exercise. Oxygen and water are key ingredients to good health. Often we need to remember how to breathe more deeply and fully. Most people practice shallow breathing out of habit. Deep healing breaths are extremely beneficial, and coupled with good water intake can help to minimize toxicity.

There are those that make the argument that the vegetables are sprayed and shot up with just as many hormones as the meat. I only know what my experience has been, in comparison to some of those who have not been as blessed. I am glad to have had this experience. Green foods and live vegetables, preferably organic vegetables and fruits, can be eaten in order to maintain proper PH balance. PH is the ratio of alkaline to acid in the bloodstream. It has been shown that when the body is slightly more alkaline that it is much less likely to breed disease. If you ever had any fish in a tank, or a pool or the like, you know the importance of maintaining proper PH balance so as to not allow fungus and other bacteria to proliferate. The human body is the same. The acid, like that found in soda, coffee, salt and other foods, make our bodies more acidic creating fertile ground for disease. PH can be measured simply in either saliva or urine with very inexpensive PH papers found in a medical supply house. Taking control of your own life can be simple. The challenge is to just do it.

The other part of having discipline in my diet has been the freedom that it has created. That is another paradox, of sorts. Until recently, it was much more of a chore to be vegetarian. When I first started living a vegetarian lifestyle, I had to look harder for a meal that fit my diet. It was not the fact that I was not eating meat that was the biggest challenge. It was more challenging to find food without eggs or egg whites in it. The freedom was created because I was not a slave to society or even my own desires. I save a great deal of money up front by the meat that I do not buy, and even more on the back end because I do not get sick. Even if I did fall ill, as I rarely have, it is because I am out of balance in some way and I am more likely brought back into balance than someone who is a meat eater.

It is another way of creating space between who I am now and the way I used to live. It has taken me more time to develop the attitude where my lifestyle is all done from a place of love instead of fear. I can now say that I love the way I live and I love the experiences that made these choices more intense.

I like to supplement my diet with herbs, vitamins and natural remedies. I get massages regularly from loving and sensitive therapist. I am not a doctor, of course, but I have come a long way towards self-empowerment. When I was diagnosed back in 1987, I was a lot more intimidated by the apparent lack of knowledge, and how much I would have to learn. It seemed like everyone else I had to go to for information knew so much more than I did. It has been a one-day at a time proposition, and over time I have become the one that people have come to for information. Most people have been watching my lifestyle and eating habits with a discriminating eye. Many have questioned, challenged and even ridiculed my eating habits. I do not engage in arguments or controversy about how I eat; I recognize that most people wanted to change their nutritional habits, but they are addicted to meat and the other things that we eat. A lot of what we eat does not serve us well, nor does it serve the universe. Some people get paid handsomely to convince us that the American diet is good. Doctors, insurance and many other parts of the economic system are dependent on people's belief that what we are eating is fine. Well, we are what we eat. Enough said about that.

I am sure that a change in diet creates more calm and rational behavior. Enhanced nutrition and conscious living can rectify some of the diabetes, attention deficit and other illnesses. Many of those same people who were either critical or just curious have begun to reconcile themselves with a change in diet. Many are changing because of physical illnesses. All of them thank me, in one way or the other, for persevering. I thank God for the courage to stick to this lifestyle. Seeing others transition and participate in their own well being is thanks enough.

GETTING INFORMATION

I have been blessed to have gotten the kind of information that has allowed me to grow. There are some books that I have read that have been instrumental in my personal shifts. *The Celestine Prophecy* spoke to the adventure of life and opened my mind to the journey's the mind can take when reading. *Conversation With God* was the book that lent more credence to things that I had been attempting to live by. To read words that verify and enhance one's deepest feelings has the effect of creating the space for change. Rich Dad, Poor Dad has encouraged me to engage life and build wealth as a way of breaking the cycle of financial limitations. There have been many helpful books.

Twelve-step literature has been integral knowledge to my personal growth. I have read a good amount of "spiritual" literature. With the further advent of the Internet, we are able to access whatever information is available on the planet. I have taught myself different trades and hobbies that have turned into passions and professions. Stimulating the mind with knowledge is key to good mental health. It helps keep us busy and minimizes the time we have for destructive mental patterns.

Having a lot of money is not mandatory to maintaining good health, but it surely makes it easier to practice healthy habits. People often say that Magic Johnson has survived with the virus because he is rich and can buy the best of everything.

I had the chance to meet Magic briefly and he plainly said that that was not the case. I am sure that having money can be beneficial, but it would not be so if one did not change their daily regimen. Medications, like the same ones that Magic, myself and millions of others have taken are only going to be maximally effective when taken in conjunction with good habits. Having said that, I have had money in my life and more often than not, have had enough money to meet my needs with much juggling and creative financing. It is much better to have money, not only for what you can buy, but for the stress that it relieves to not have to worry about if you can pay your bills. Having good financial health is a result of many things, but is a manifestation of attitude and how well we implement certain universal principles. Having the virus has affected my moods and attitude even as I practice positivism. Counseling has proved to be helpful in helping me to shift from attitudes and behaviors that caused me to create periods of lack.

During the course of writing this book I experienced a metamorphosis of my own. My family has gone through a very profound transition as well. Before I started writing this book I had not disclosed my HIV positive status to anyone other than my wife. I had not told my mother, sister, any of my four children, any other relatives or friends. I had not publicly acknowledged my status for the previous 15 years of my journey. I credit my sister with having the courage to ask me the question about my status after one of my visits to New York where she and much of my family still reside. I had lost weight due to another condition called hyperthyroidism and she was alarmed and concerned. I did not know how weak and fragile I was looking as the condition caused me to lose a great deal of weight. I am 6'4" and my usual weight is 175 pounds. I had gotten down to 149 pounds and my wife was scared to death that she was going to lose me. Although Dionne is sometimes more dramatic than I would consider necessary, she had a legitimate concern. My sister and many others apparently were concerned as well, but people never tell you how bad you look until you start improving. When Pam asked me straight up what the deal was, I told her. We had the conversation by phone, and as usual, my sister provided love and support. She also provided a sense of relief that I had been wanting unconsciously. I did not think that my not talking about my diagnosis was a secret even though I was not talking about it at all with anyone. It was just my own dilemma and I did not think my family or the world was capable of being of any assistance; I felt it would just worry them about something they could do absolutely nothing about. I did not want to worry my children or especially my mother. I wanted to protect them all, as well as myself, from the negative energy that I felt would be the result of disclosure.

After beginning my family's journey of disclosure, I attained a new freedom that I did not expect. My newfound freedom caused major changes in the dynamic between Dionne and myself, because for the first time in 15 years my disclosing caused us to have to deal more honestly with my having the virus. Moreover, we had to deal with her negative status and how people were going to perceive what we had been through. There are many people who had to really think about some of the things they may have said or done not knowing that I was HIV positive and living with full-blown AIDS for all of these years. Mainly, Dionne had trouble dealing with the scrutiny. I was compelled to tell my story. I was motivated by the response that I got from strangers I met at the IBI Forum, a networking opportunity where I learned of my true wealth from Joel Roberts, media coach extraordinaire. That experience changed me and helped me to see that it may help a great number of people if we shared what we have been through. We could be granted the serenity to accept the things we could not change, the courage to change the things we could, and the wisdom to know the difference, we would being living in God's will and further surrendering to what is. I had no idea the level of healing that was available on the other side. I cannot say that I did not have some intuition about needing to be able to speak freely about what my personal truth is. I had wanted to be more honest about my life for years. What we were doing was working relatively well, so I did not want to upset my family and change the energy I had tried my best to maintain at all cost. When I was granted the blessing of my wife and later from the rest of my family, I was set free. Not coincidentally, my doctor, Dr. William Richardson, diagnosed my thyroid issue, and not long after that, the condition has been stabilized. I am hovering around 170 pounds now and that is fine with me. I have been blessed to have continued good health and for that I thank God.

As I began to write this book, I realized that I would now have to tell my mother what our situation was. I know how much my mother loves me and I did not want to have to cause her any worry or stress about me. I was very happy that even though we had lost my father many years ago, my mother had had the chance to see me get and stay clean, to be a father, son and friend to those that love me, and to pursue my dreams. I am most happy for that dream. I knew that I needed to tell her at some point before we were able to speak publicly because I did not want her to hear it from someone else. It was one of the hardest things that I ever have done. I rode to New York for Christmas in 2002 determined to have the conversation before I left the city. It had already been months since I had told the kids and my sister, and I was beginning to be much more active as an advocate. I became intent on changing the way that this disease is perceived and portrayed.

I knew it would hit my mother hard and she was devastated in a caring and dignified way. As I broached the topic, my mother's intuition kicked in and she finished my sentence for me. It seems she had been curious about it and had a sense that I had come to New York this time with a purpose. She later said that she knew I had something to tell her. My mother is very strong and she has quickly adapted as well as she can. She suffered some serious physical challenges months after I told her, but as scary as that was I am glad to have seen her make a full recovery. I would have hated to think that my desire to be free, to be me and to attempt to help others, would have a negative impact on my own mother. I did not want my own freedom at her expense. Thank God all is well, just for today. The relationship between my mother and myself is better than ever before. We had already begun to do some of the healing work needed to help us get past resentments held for a very long time, and I think that has helped our entire family to be able to heal. I have been open to, and have practiced information from traditions outside of my experience. They have been the traditions and practices that have rung true in my heart. We all have to find that with which we resonate. My experience has been that more has been revealed as I have become prepared for it. I might never have been in India, sitting at the feet of my guru, had it not been for the things that had come before it. I would not have been as open to an education about quantum physics and quantum mechanics, where I learned about the mind and some of its vast ability, had I not been exposed to the Path. I may not have had the awareness to put principles before personalities had it not been for the experiences that came before that teaching. Contempt prior to investigation breeds everlasting ignorance.

EVOLUTION

It has been a process learning to love others and myself. My wife and I are both in recovery and doing the best that we could to share whatever blessings we have had with other addicts and alcoholics. As of this writing, she has been diagnosed as being not infected and for that I am truly grateful. She has been courageous beyond what I could have asked or imagined. She has supported me in ways that I am eternally grateful for. When I was too depressed to work or want to interact, she was the thread that I clung to. Though we did the best we could to not live in the problem, the situation had a profound effect on our family's lives and ours. Not necessarily in an overt way, but it colored the decisions we have made in a definite way. Without my wife to go through my life, I would have most certainly experienced more strife.

There are a few things that I believe to be essential in the process of healing from this or any other disease. One is faith in a Higher Power, a loving God as he may express himself in your life. That faith allowed me to tap into a power greater than myself. That power has relieved me of many addictions, their compulsions and obsessions and delivered me thus far into freedom. Without that Power I do not know where I would be. Probably dead, I imagine.

Faith, though, does not relieve us of the responsibility of "participating in our own survival." We need evaluate, with the help of physicians, herbalists, and many of the other healing modalities, a path and course of action that will serve us best—and then we must live it. There are so many people that know what they should be doing in order to have the best quality of life. Besides the motivation of wanting to be in good health, there need be a sense of responsibility to our loved ones to put up the best defense. I have now learned the value of having the opportunity to be honest about who we truly are. The stigma surrounding this disease of AIDS has certainly contributed to far too many premature deaths, if there is such a thing as a premature death. No one is going to get out of this thing alive, I always say. Being honest about who I am has been powerful for everyone, specifically myself. Having the conversation about participating in one's own survival is at the core of a movement I find myself a part of. Many people have come, and some have gone, having succumbed to the challenges of these diseases. Many people worked hard to make it possible for me to be alive and to even want to have the courage to be of service. I honor and salute them for what they did to combat the stigma of drug addiction, alcoholism and AIDS, and fight for the funding for research and treatment. They did so facing fear and discrimination while making it possible for me to be about the business of raising my children. I was blessed to be carrying the message of hope in many ways, but I was not talking about being infected. I applaud the courage and determination of those who have fought and died on the battlefields of life. May God bless them all. This book is an example that anything is possible and there is hope for all of us. Together we can. If I am blessed to do so, I would like to be a part of helping to create the environment that will be conducive to having the conversation about how to participate in your own survival.

Love has been the bedrock of my salvation. I have been

blessed to find love in many places, none more important, consistent, understanding and tolerant than my wife. Even if you do not feel comfortable sharing your particular situation with many—or any—you should have at least one or two people that you are close enough to share with. I only really had my wife until recently coming out and sharing with many. It has been a process for me, that is still evolving, but I am happier being able to be more honest. It has allowed me to write this book, something that I have been compelled to do for some time now.

Curiosity is something that motivates me as well. I am very interested in seeing how things are going to turn out in 200 years. Some folks say they would not want to be around that long, but that is with the understanding that their bodies would deteriorate with time. I believe that, like Jack LaLanne, Methuselah and my historically ancient cultures, long periods of life can be had if we can take care of our bodies so that they can take care of us. Exercise, sunshine and fresh air are essential for the healing. I had stopped playing basketball competitively for over ten years or more before making a comeback for the past two and a half years. At the age of 47, I am working out, swimming, biking, playing basketball and softball and doing them on a really respectable level. I feel really good about it, and that is a part of the healing process.

Tapping into your passion for life helps give you direction. When we are able to identify what Gods gifts are for us, and how they show up in our lives, we are able to listen to the voice within. That is, more often than not, the path to personal enlightenment. Just like Dorothy and her crew in the Wizard Of Oz, follow the yellow brick road. Just like in that prophetic drama, the search for courage, heart and knowledge will culminate in self.

Living the dream is really important. Go for it. What the hell have you got to lose? It is certain that my experience has helped me realize the "courage to change the things that I can...." When you think that there is a possibility that life may soon end, you internalize the "one day at a time" concept more easily. That is a much more beneficial attitude than to think yourself into martyrdom. I almost did that, and I will tell you that living the dream is much more fun. When you are facing your own mortality, you get a chance to test your faith. I have had to stand for what I acknowledged as being truth, sometimes in the face of logic and common knowledge contrary to what I chose to have faith in. I thank God for the test of faith, and for the courage to grow through those choices and situations.

My dream is one of freedom. Free to be whoever I want to be. Free to give love and be loved. Free to live life to the best of my ability. Being drug free was the beginning of my being free. Quitting smoking and refraining from eating meat has helped me to increase my level of freedom.

When I started to think about what I really needed, which we are prone to do when we think we might die, I realized that I did not really need that much. Love, food, water, clothing and shelter are among the priorities. When the new millennium came around, I was one of the people who was preparing for the worst. I had been getting in the prepared state of mind even before that. The reason is that I want to be free. If I have the ability to build a house for my family, and myself to grow food and to survive without the pressure of our own desires, we have created a personal freedom for ourselves.

Here is where the adventure gets good. The thought of wanting to be free has been manifest once again. I thought about building a log cabin totally off the grid. My vision was/is to build a log cabin with solar energy, geothermal heat, air and hot water, potbellied stove, etc.. I thought about having some land of our own to build it on, rural land away from the hustle and bustle. I wanted a place to create an atmosphere of peace. All of these dreams are being manifest now as we are in the planning stage of building the cabin on some rural land that was recently divided within my family.

This will give me the opportunity to continue to do some of the healing with my ancestors. I have been learning more about my ancestors and it has served as a form of healing. I believe that by helping my mother to deal with a resentment that she did not take the opportunity to resolve in over 60 years, I am helping not only her. I believe that that healing will transcend time and generations. I can see how it is healing children, my grandchildren and me.

"...We must become like little children..."

In order to evolve we must stay open minded. Children have less problem with being honest and speaking their minds. It gets tricky when we have to start to learn what emotions are and then begin to want to protect our feelings. We become dishonest when we worry about what we are going to lose, or what we are not going to get. Desires have the ability to imprison us in our minds. It does not matter whether our fetters are made of iron or gold: both enslave us.

The trick is to find the proper balance. I still enjoy luxury and I am moving to create an environment that includes much luxury. I have been learning to put in the effort to obtain these things, but not be tied emotionally to the outcome of the effort. The better I get at this delicate balance, the quicker these things manifest. It is also part of universal law. I do not know if this book will help anyone else going through anything close to the same kind of situation. I certainly hope so. I do know that I give these words in loving service. In doing so, there is great relief. I truly feel that it serves me better to not retreat from my reality, but to share it. Where that will lead me, I am excited to watch. I always say, "I enjoy watching the adventure of life unfold." I am very excited about the possibilities. My plan is to continue to do my best to help God use me for whatever. I wish the same for you.

The Father, Son, Holy Spirit is a Holy Trinity. It is reflected in the thought, word and deed. Everything begins with a thought. What we say is soon manifest in who we are to be. The art of being in the present enhances how we live. Not being consumed by the past or the future keeps the present in our consciousness.

There are no words to express my gratitude for the opportunity to fulfill this destiny. The God in me salutes the God in you. If you had not been destined to read this book, I would not have been destined to live and write it. Everything happens for a reason. I am grateful to the Creator in you for making my life possible and valuable. God loves you, and I do too.

THE CHAKRA SYSTEM

FIRST CHAKRA: Area of the Body: Organs of Elimination
HUMAN TALENT: Acceptance
COLOR: Red
SHADOW EMOTION(S): Resentment, Rigidity
ELEMENT: Earth

SECOND CHAKRA: Area of the Body: The Sexual Organs
HUMAN TALENT: Creativity
COLOR: Orange
SHADOW EMOTION(S): Passionate manipulation, Guilt
ELEMENT: Water

THIRD CHAKRA: Area of the Body: Navel Center
HUMAN TALENT: Commitment
COLOR: Yellow Shadow
EMOTION(S): Anger, Greed
ELEMENT: Fire

FOURTH CHAKRA : Area of the Body: Heart Center
HUMAN TALENT: Compassion
COLOR: Green Shadow

EMOTION(S): Fear, Attachment
ELEMENT: Air

FIFTH CHAKRA: Area of the Body: Throat
HUMAN TALENT: Truth
COLOR: Blue Shadow
EMOTION(S): Denial, Abruptness
ELEMENT: Ether

SIXTH CHAKRA: Area of the Body: Third Eye Point
HUMAN TALENT: Intuition
COLOR: Indigo
SHADOW EMOTION(S): Confusion, Depression
ELEMENT: None

SEVENTH CHAKRA: Area of the Body: Crown of the Head
HUMAN TALENT: Boundlessness
COLOR: Violet
SHADOW EMOTION(S) : Grief
ELEMENT: None

EIGHTH CHAKRA: Area of the Body: The Electromagnetic Field (Aura)
HUMAN TALENT: Radiance
COLOR: White
SHADOW EMOTION(S) : None
ELEMENT: None

You will notice that the first five chakras are each associated with an earthly element—earth, water, fire, air, and ether. Most people recognize the first four elements, but are unfamiliar with the term "ether." Ether is a subtle, heavenly energy, beyond the earth. As we move up the ladder of chakras, into the higher mental and spiritual realms, there are no longer earthly elements associated with these chakras. Lust, anger, greed, pride, and attachment are human qualities that result from the imbalance of the eight energy centers called chakras. When these imbalances settle in, we often experience mental or physical problems.

People often come to me with emotional blocks in a certain chakra that have manifested in the creation of a physical illness. The idea that certain emotions and talents live in certain areas of our bodies is not a new one, but I do think some people have taken this too far, and assume that if they get sick it is somehow their own fault. This is a negative way of looking at this phenomenon, and does more harm than good when it comes to healing our bodies and spirits. Your disease is not your fault. Illness is part of the whole learning experience of life, and everybody goes through it. That's what it means to be mortal. You can take an active, positive role in healing your own mind, body, and spirit.

***

See your body as God's perfect gift to you, for it is in loving and appreciating our body that we begin the path to consciousness. The eight greatest talents of humankind are located in the eight chakras, the eight major power areas of the body. The Eight Human Talents are the gifts of God that make us different from all other creatures on earth. Happiness is your birthright. The use and cultivation of these eight talents are keys to the happiness that God wants for you.

Happiness is your birthright.

Our bodies are gifts from God. We need them to be here.

For it is in loving and appreciating our bodies that we begin the path to consciousness. Happiness is your birthright. Opening, or balancing all your chakras is the key to that happiness.

> "The very purpose of our life is happiness, the very motion of our life is towards happiness."
> —The Dalai Lama

It's nearly impossible to balance these eight power centers perfectly to bring out their talents every day of your life. But don't worry; perfection isn't the goal. The goal is to become aware of the energy emanating from each chakra and to be able to call upon it when you need it. Let's say you're called on to make a presentation at a board meeting. You'll need to shift into the fifth chakra located at your throat to communicate your ideas clearly, and the third chakra to give your presentation the special emphasis and punch of commitment. If an angry coworker blows up over the smallest inconvenience, don't meet fire with fire. Try meeting her with your fourth chakra, using compassion to heal the fear and insecurity behind her outburst.

Our bodies are like complex worlds within worlds. We know where they begin and end, and yet they are vast and full of mysteries that we may never understand. No machine has ever been devised by a human that is as complex or artful as our own human body. The ancient system of chakras is a way to understand ourselves. There is an incredible amount of subtle interaction going on all the time.

I have chosen specific Kundalini Yoga exercise sequences and meditations to help you develop the human talent that lies hidden within each chakra. I suggest you choose one or two, and try them for three minutes at least. I always suggest that students begin trying any meditation for three minutes, and increase it to seven, then eleven, eventually working up to thirty-one minutes. You can see improvement by committing to doing the meditation for a longer period of time.

"The life of a yogi is to manifest a beautiful, bountiful and wonderfully blissful tomorrow. That's a yogi."
—Yogi Bhajan

The reason for these specific lengths of time has to do with the numerological significance of each number in the Kundalini Yoga tradition. The greater the amount of time spent in meditation, the greater the benefit. In Kundalini Yoga, we often do movements twenty-six times. Because we have twenty-six vertebrae, twenty-six is an important number to us. For a greater challenge, you can increase the number of repetitions of an exercise to fifty-four or even one hundred and eight if you really want to see faster progress!

It's not what you do, but the courage and commitment that you bring to what you do.

Meditation is not about perfecting or attaining anything. People think they need to go into a trance or be in an altered state to feel they're really meditating. That can and does happen, but meditation is actually the clearinghouse of the mind. Our minds release a thousand thoughts per wink of the eye. Just watch these thoughts as you might watch an ocean wave, not remembering or diagnosing them as they come and go. The real gift is to sit in the middle of all those thoughts, and react to not a one. Keep returning back to your breath, or maybe the sound you're making or the position of your body.

Kundalini Meditations usually consist of breath or sound patterns and some specific positions, so you have plenty on which to concentrate.

"Each thought can become an emotion, and a feeling. And with each emotion and feeling, some of them become desires, and to be completed they take up all of your life energy. But if you use every thought and pass it through the intelligence and test it with your consciousness, you shall be successful, doesn't matter what. That's a simple secret of life."
—Yogi Bhajan

When there's an emergency—for example, if someone is calling from a hospital—we'll say, "Okay, take a deep breath, and slow down." When you don't allow yourself to breathe, you deny yourself the very gift of life. In yogic terms, we believe that the life force is the "prana," which comes to us through the breath. Allowing yourself to take in enough breath is usually the first thing you need, and it's usually the first thing to go. Breath is free for the taking, but we're often very miserly in the way we dole it out to ourselves. It's not logical, but we all do it.

Before I learned this particular technology for meditation, I experienced the frustration of being told to sit and "meditate," having no idea what that meant. I'm so glad that I now have specific tools and techniques that make meditation less mysterious and more practical.

If you want to make a real change and develop the talent in any chakra, I suggest you do a meditation for that power center for forty days, for whatever length of time feels comfortable. You can start with a shorter time and then increase the time during the forty-day period. If you just aren't up to it one day, you can go back to a three-minute period for that day so you don't have to break your forty-day commitment.

Forty days has historically been a significant time period in many world religions. In the Old Testament it rained for forty days and forty nights. In Christianity there are the forty days of Lent. Forty-day cycles are very important in the Sikh religion as well. Perhaps this is because your physical body renews all the cells in your bloodstream every forty days. For whatever reason, forty days has always been a mystical period of time.

So you see, there are many ways to use these tools. I don't want you ever to feel that the one you pick is not good enough. It doesn't matter if you do something for three minutes or for thirty-one minutes—it's all good. In this work, it is not what you do, but the focus and depth you bring to it.

Of course, it is my deepest prayer that after you do this work even on the smallest level, you will see real improvement in your life, and you will be inspired to devote more time to using these life-changing tools. In a lifetime of teaching, I have seen the practice of Yoga and Meditation create miracles of healing. If you want healing on any level of your life and you are willing to do the work, you will see miracles, too.

The first chakra, which contains the human talent of acceptance, encompasses our organs of elimination. Here we find foundation, security, and habit. The second chakra, which contains our reproductive organs, is where we find the human talent of creativity. In the third chakra, we come to the solar plexus area, the stomach, and many of the internal organs, such as the liver and the spleen. This area is the center for energy, for world power, for a sense of control and coordination. It is ruled by the element of fire.

Of these chakras—the first, second, and third, which make up what we call the lower triangle—the third is the subtlest. It is the driving force to act and to complete the conceptualization, the visualization that we have in our lives. It is where we find the human talent of commitment. In the heart center, the fourth chakra, we find compassion. The throat area, the fifth chakra, is the part of the body in which we literally "find our voice." This chakra houses the human talent of truth.

The sixth chakra is classically located at the point between the eyebrows, which yogis refer to as the "third eye point," and contains intuition. This is where we find our sense of physical vision, and our extrasensory talent of vision as well. The seventh chakra is located at the top of the head. The exact area is where the tiny endocrine organ, known as the pineal gland, is found near the crown of the head, where the soft spot on a newborn baby's head is located. This chakra contains the human talent of boundlessness. It is the spiritual center of our physical body. This experience of boundlessness has many names in many world religions. I chose the word "boundlessness" to describe this spiritual connection, without the specific association of any particular religion.

The last chakra encompasses what is referred to in yogic science as the electromagnetic field. It is our aura, a field of energy surrounding our physical body that makes up the eighth chakra. Western science has proved the existence of this field as a physical phenomenon. The human talent that lives in this chakra is that of radiance. As you can see, each energy center has a profound impact on our lives. At any given time, we may lose touch with one or another of them, become imbalanced and feel "off." The purpose of this book is to find ways to connect, strengthen, and balance each of these centers on a daily basis. This process is sometimes referred to as "balancing the chakras." It is the very purpose of our lives; it is a constant and worthwhile process.

"If you ever want to be right in your life, bring yourself into balance. The joy of life, the happiness of life, is in balance."
—Yogi Bhajan

***

When we are unbalanced in our chakras or energy centers, we use those expressions like, "I'm having an off day," "I'm having a bad hair day," "Nothing seemed to go right today." If the chakras are balanced, you'll hear expressions like, "It was such a great day," "It was such a miraculous day. Things went so smoothly today!" And that comes when everything is lined up and the energy is flowing throughout your whole body. Yoga is the science of breath and angles. It is an ancient science, put together by our wise elders, who were in tune with the energy field of the universe and how it manifests through our physical bodies. When we study yoga, we learn to place our arms, hands, and fingers, and the body itself into very specific postures, creating certain angles. Combined with powerful breathing techniques, these postures can produce amazing changes in our psyche!

"Before us the sages have laid the path. We are taking our first step."
—Yogi Bhajan

Yoga is similar to what keeps most animals fit. One only has to watch the stretching exercises that a cat does, and then see her magnificent body in action as she chases a bird, to understand that the systematic stretching and relaxation of our muscles can keep us fit for life.

In our uniquely human capacity to connect movement with breath and spiritual meaning, yoga is born. The translation of the word "yoga" is " union." This union of breath and movement has as its ultimate goal the harmonious merging of body, mind, and soul into the universal energy surrounding us. We refer to it as the "practice of yoga," and that is what we do in the Yoga classes. But the real yoga is how you take what you've learned in class and live it out in the world.

People who are new to yoga ask me, "Is it hard? Do I have to be some kind of athlete?" Oftentimes, they give up on the very idea of yoga before they've even tried it, because they assume that it is something that dancers and acrobats do. I have students who are world-class athletes, and students who are amputees, or paraplegics, or cardiac rehab patients. Absolutely anyone can do this yoga, and everyone will be challenged by it, too. And everyone I have ever seen attempt it, even on the smallest level, has been changed. But please, if you have a medical condition, consult your doctor or chiropractor if you are unsure if your body is ready for a new challenge. Yogic technology is not a substitute for medical advice or attention; one needs to be sensitive when dealing with the complexities of the body. Once you are aware of your limitations, then be sensitive and get going!

As to "Is it hard?"—yes, it is. Sometimes it's physically hard, sometimes it just annoys a part of your mind, what we sometimes call the "Monkey Mind." The Monkey Mind is the part of your mind that doesn't want to consider the higher questions of life. While the monkey might be asking, "Where is my next banana?" the human is asking, "Where's the next doughnut, cigarette, or mocha latte?" And the Monkey Mind will lie to you, to make sure you keep the bananas or the mocha lattes coming its way. It will tell you that this yoga you are doing is tedious, pointless, silly. Your Monkey Mind can make the yoga seem harder than it is, because it doesn't want to change.

So our Monkey Mind will tell us to turn away from things like yoga, things that portend change and seem "hard." I think we are at a point in history at which we want things to come easily. We have come to value easiness. We want a pill that will fix everything. We just want it taken care of, we want to be fixed, and we want it now. We want our lives to be pain-free, and the lives of our children to be pain-free. But what are we really looking for when we try a new diet or a new drug or a new religion? We get discouraged when things aren't easy and perfect. Yoga can be challenging, but unlike a painkiller, its purpose isn't to mask our pain. It heals our pain. Yogi Bhajan has said

"There is no freedom which is free."

I know, because I have been that person seeking. I spent a great deal of my life searching for the easy, pain-free fix. In my early twenties, I became addicted to heroin and cocaine, because that seemed like the pain-free path to freedom. Of course, it was not. Pain is part of the deal.

When I think back to that time, I was so sure someone must have the answer. I wanted someone to tell me how to make my life pain-free. Looking back, I can't imagine who I thought got through their entire lives and managed to avoid the pain. Now I realize there is not now nor has there ever been a single person on this planet who has successfully avoided the pain of being human. Pain is part of the deal.

In fact, the enlightened beings who have graced this

planet dealt with the pain of humanness, and it is usually the main point of their story. This is true with Jesus, with Buddha, with Moses, with Gandhi. How did I think I could get around it?

Now since I accept pain as part of the human bargain, I am also free to accept the serenity I believe is my natural state of being. God wants each of us to live in a state of serenity. Serenity, which encompasses happiness and joy, also allows for pain and sorrow, because serenity is a state of being that accepts all of our states without judgment. Serenity is the state of being that exists when we are in balance, when we know our place in the universe, when we are truly able to accept God's will for us. It was the study of Yoga and Meditation that taught me about balance and serenity, taught me how to quiet my chattering Monkey Mind, taught me how to focus on and be grateful for each breath I take. Yoga and Meditation have helped me to re-pattern my body and my mind.

As I began to learn this yoga, I began to escape the illusion I could or even wanted to avoid pain. I did begin to see pain, discomfort, and even simple annoyance, as the learning opportunities and blessings that they are. I still don't always see the traffic jam as "a growth opportunity." At first, unconsciously, I may mistake it for a complaining opportunity. And then sometimes the traffic jam, or the grocery line, or any other daily test sends me directly into impatience. I start thinking about whose fault it is that I'm stuck in traffic, or how I shouldn't have to be dealing with this. Yoga and Meditation have helped me to re-pattern my body and my mind, so that I don't stay in the illusion of "why me" quite as long, and even when I'm in it, I remember "this too shall pass."

This yoga can be challenging, but it can also bring peace. Once you get past the pain or the discomfort or even the simple annoyance, there can be such bliss and joy in the breath and the movement. Someone sent me a story on the Internet that so perfectly summed up this paradox of how challenging experiences make us stronger.

One day a small opening appeared on a cocoon, and a man sat and watched for the butterfly for several hours as it struggled to force its body through that little hole. Then it seemed to stop making any progress. It appeared as if it had gotten as far as it could and it could go no further.

So the man decided to help the butterfly. He took a pair of scissors and snipped off the remaining bit of the cocoon. The butterfly then emerged easily. But it had a swollen body and small, shriveled wings. The man continued to watch the butterfly because he expected that, at any moment, the wings would enlarge and expand to be able to support the body, which would contract in time. Neither happened!

In fact, the butterfly spent the rest of its life crawling around with a swollen body and shriveled wings. It never was able to fly.

What the man, in his kindness and haste, did not understand was that the restricting cocoon and the struggle required for the butterfly to get through the tiny opening was God's way of forcing fluid from the body of the butterfly into its wings so that it would be ready for flight once it achieved its freedom from the cocoon.

Sometimes struggles are exactly what we need in our life. If God allowed us to go through our life without any obstacles, it would cripple us. We would not be as strong as we could have been. We could never fly.

I asked for Strength ...
And God gave me Challenges to make me strong.

I asked for Wisdom ...
And God gave me Problems to solve.
I asked for Prosperity ...
And God gave me Brain and Brawn to work.
I asked for Courage ...
And God gave me Danger to overcome.
I asked for Love ...
And God gave me Troubled people to help.
I asked for Favors ...
And God gave me Opportunities.
I received nothing I wanted
I received everything I needed.

I asked God for a way to avoid pain, and God gave me opportunities. Know that each of these eight energy centers already lives within you, each of the chakras is like that butterfly trying to be born out of its cocoon. The whole process of learning is really the process of uncovering and rediscovering what we already know. That is the process we will undergo together. I know by the end of this journey we will see our eight glorious human talents begin to thrive. We humans are magnificent creatures. This is the perfect time for us to celebrate and nurture our Eight Human Talents together. Our bodies are the means by which we come to know and understand our spiritual connection to the Infinite. John O'Donohue, gifted poet of the spirit, sums up this relationship beautifully in the Celtic poem from his book *Anam Cara: A Book of Celtic Wisdom—A Blessing For The Senses*

May your body be blessed.
May you realize that your body is a faithful and
beautiful friend of your soul.

And may you be peaceful and joyful and recognize
that your senses are sacred thresholds.
May you realize that holiness is mindful, gazing,
feeling, hearing, and touching.
May your senses gather you and bring you home.
May your senses always enable you to celebrate the universe
and the mystery and possibilities in your presence here.
May the Eros of the Earth bless you

With Permission Copyright © 2000 Gurmukh with Cathryn Michon

Here I would like to refer to some of the books I have read.

The Power of Now by Ekhart Tolle

Conversation with God (books 1,2,3), *Communion with God* by Neale Donald Walsh

Kabir by V.K. Setthe

The Four Agreements by Don Miguel Ruiz

The *Big Books* of Alcoholic Anonymous and Narcotics Anonymous

The HIV Anonymous Workbook—

Principles of the Spirit by Glen Caulkins

For more information on the HIV Anonymous 12-step program please visit www.hivanonymous.com

The Path of the Masters by Julian Johnson

A Matter of Time by Don Kirchner

Also, anything written by Deepak Chopra is most beneficial to expanding one's scope and enhancing our human experience.

For more information on books and other resources that

have been effective for myself and others in our quest for wholeness, please visit our website at www.sameboat.tv

The Five Divine Senses
        by Debi Smith

Awareness (I AM)
Imagination (Creation)
Compassion (Unity and Togetherness)
Focus (Power)—blend imagination and compassion to create reality
Expression—using energies to birth creation
LOVE...what you GIVE is what you LIVE!!
BREATHE in and BREATHE out LIGHT AND LOVE daily